Turmeric

Turmeric

Nature's Miracle Healer:
Fact or Fiction?

PENELOPE ODY

Souvenir Press

In memory of Ernest Hecht
whose idea initiated this book

First published in Great Britain in 2018 by Souvenir Press Ltd
43 Great Russell Street, London WC1B 3PD

ISBN 9780285644038

Typeset by M Rules

Printed and bound in Great Britain
by CPI Group (UK) Ltd, Croydon, CR0 4YY

Note to Readers

The aim of this book is to provide a balanced view of the potential medical applications of turmeric and its derivatives in the light of recent research – both positive and negative. It neither endorses nor censures any of the commercial products mentioned in its pages. In the UK, products based on turmeric or its derivatives, unless prescribed by a healthcare professional, are sold only as food supplements so cannot claim to deliver any specific medical benefits.

Where health is concerned   and in particular for a serious problem of any kind – it must be stressed that there is no substitute for seeking advice from a qualified healthcare professional rather than attempting self-medication based on Internet or other sources. It is important, if you are already taking prescribed medication and are considering trying food supplements based on turmeric or its derivatives, that you consult your healthcare practitioner first. If you experience any unexpected symptoms when taking turmeric or its derivatives, it is advisable to stop immediately and seek professional advice.

The Publisher makes no representation, express or implied

with regard to the accuracy of the information contained in this book, and legal responsibility or liability cannot be accepted by the Author or Publisher for any errors or omissions that may be made or for any loss, damage, injury or problems suffered in anyway arising from following any advice offered in these pages.

Contents

Chapter 1

Fashionable hype . . . and confusion

One of those irritating spam e-mails arriving in my in-box just as I began writing this book seemed to sum it all up perfectly: Turmeric *". . . a remedy for every kind of human inflammation, [brand name] now brings it to you in a bottle! CURES WHATEVER AILS YOU. If you talk to turmeric fans, they'll tell you it can cure cancer, reduce your risk of disease, and flood your body with life-saving anti-oxidants"*.

The spam message was typical of the advertising that surrounds many of the turmeric-based remedies sold in health food shops. If even half the marketing hype one reads about turmeric were true it could well fall into the "nature's miracle" category. The question to ask is, of course, just how valid are the numerous claims made for the herb? Traditionally, turmeric's medicinal uses have been far more limited than much of the current media hype suggests. If it really achieves half the cures claimed for it, then it would be rather strange if these actions had only become apparent in the past 20 years and had never been noticed during its millennia of use. Perhaps the "placebo effect" is playing a part with those "turmeric fans" so convinced of the herb's near-magical properties that the health benefits they perceive are a classic case of mind over matter?

Turmeric – particularly its chemical constituents, the curcuminoids, responsible for the yellow colouring – has been extensively studied in recent decades. In 2015 a database[1] was established to attempt to keep track of all this research. At the time of writing it lists 10,971 publications on curcumin as well as 962 patents involving the substance.

An extensive review of curcumin chemistry published in 2017[2] noted that since the late 1990s the number of scientific papers published about curcumin had increased exponentially from around 100 per year to some 1,400 in 2016. Although this study focussed on curcumin chemistry, rather than turmeric as a whole, it noted how any negative studies about the constituent tended to be "swept away" in the face of a ". . . torrent of papers, reviews, patents, and Websites touting the use of curcumin . . . as an anticancer agent, a therapeutic for Alzheimer's disease, a treatment for hangovers, erectile dysfunction, baldness, hirsutism, a fertility-boosting and contraceptive extract, collectively establishing the properties expected of a panacea". While the curcuminoids have been the focus of much research, this study raised significant questions as to whether these chemicals really are entirely responsible for turmeric's therapeutic properties. Not that this appears to concern the manufacturers of the various curcumin extracts.

Much research into herbs is aimed at identifying key chemical constituents, which can then be individually extracted or replicated synthetically to produce unique "drugs". These can be patented and thus become profitable for the companies involved. There is little incentive in researching – at considerable expense – a "whole" plant that can then be grown in a back garden or foraged and be used – for minimal expense – by anyone who wishes to benefit.

A problem with this isolated chemical approach is, of course, that as far as herbs are concerned the whole plant is often greater than the sum if its parts. Examples abound: such as meadowsweet (*Filipendula ulmaria*) which contains the same chemical as aspirin, but the whole herb is used as a remedy for gastritis, whereas aspirin alone is a significant cause of stomach inflammation; or dandelion leaf (*Taraxacum officinale*) – a potent diuretic – that is extremely rich in potassium, which is lost from the body by excessive urination, so the herb is effectively putting back what it is taking out.

We also know very little about how the various chemical constituents of a plant work together to create physiological effects. While the constituents of many herbs have been identified there are often a few that remain unclassified and inevitably the mix varies depending on growing conditions, age of the plant, soil composition and so on. While individual plant constituents can be highly significant – as with digoxin and digitoxin from the foxglove – when used in isolation these chemicals can have very different therapeutic properties from the "whole" plant.

The result, seen on any health food store shelf, is that while some manufacturers are happy to sell capsules filled only with turmeric powder, many others prefer to offer a variety of curcuminoid extracts: sometimes just curcumin, sometimes all of the curcuminoids, and sometimes a mixture of curcumin and other herbs or vitamins.

The various curcumin and curcuminoid extracts are produced by a small number of global companies specialising in biotechnology or pharmaceuticals (see Chapter 4). These patented products are then used by numerous supplement manufacturers to make the wide assortment of pills, capsules and liquid extracts available. The various patented products have also been used in many company-sponsored research studies and clinical trials, which are used to support the various claims made by the producers of the final consumer products.

How these manufacturers market the final products varies and can lead to significant confusion in the claims they make and the language they use to promote their products. Because curcumin has poor absorption when taken orally (most is simply excreted) the extract makers have tried various tactics to improve its "bioavailability". One website[3], for example, offers a product that "contains 95% curcuminoids" and declares that turmeric has "traditionally been used for nearly every health condition known – from smallpox to a sprained ankle". Another[4] puts its claim for a comparable product rather differently as "yields 95% curcuminoids". "Yield" is entirely different to "contains" as it implies how much of the curcuminoids present may be available to someone taking the remedy. Some talk of enhancing bioavailability by up to "285 times" while others prefer to claim "2000%", which is mathematically confusing.

The various "curcuminoid" capsules on the market typically contain anything from 20mg to 250mg or more of the designated extract and, typically, two capsules per day are recommended. The amount of curcuminoids in turmeric varies, from about 1% to 6% – occasionally more – depending on variety and where grown, but generally accepted to average about 4.5%. Given this low and variable content, if the curcuminoids really are the key therapeutic constituents high doses of turmeric would probably have been needed in the past to have any significant affect.

Doses of turmeric suggested by today's herbalists vary: the simplest will probably involve a teaspoonful of powdered rhizome (about 4g) mixed with milk to form a slurry and to be taken twice a day. This would deliver around 360mg of curcuminoids. Chinese medicine – not known for prescribing low quantities of herbs – gives the recommended dose of whole turmeric as 3–9g per day, which could provide, on average, anything from 135mg to 405mg of curcuminoids daily. These turmeric dosages thus provide rather less curcumin than that supposedly delivered by many of today's curcumin "food supplements"; in reported clinical trials involving extracts, dosages of 2–5g of curcumin daily are not uncommon.

Increasing the dosage of any herb is not always going to deliver greater benefit: it can simply increase the risk of side effects. As the 15th century herbalist Paracelsus famously declared: "In all things there is a poison and there is nothing without a poison. It depends only upon the dose whether a poison is a poison or not."

For anyone hoping to use turmeric to treat a particular ailment or improve their general health, the wide variation in curcuminoid content and apparent dosages is confusing. As is the enormous range of ailments which turmeric is said to treat. The list provided by one online health site[5] is impressive: "Turmeric is used for arthritis, heartburn (dyspepsia), joint pain, stomach pain, Crohn's disease and ulcerative colitis, bypass surgery, haemorrhage, diarrhoea, intestinal gas, stomach bloating, loss of appetite, jaundice, liver problems, *Helicobacter pylori* (H. pylori) infection, stomach ulcers, irritable bowel syndrome (IBS), gallbladder disorders, high cholesterol, lichen planus, skin inflammation from radiation treatment, fatigue, headaches, bronchitis, colds, lung infections, fibromyalgia, leprosy, fever, menstrual problems, itchy skin, recovery after surgery, cancers, depression, Alzheimer's disease, swelling in the middle layer of the eye (anterior uveitis), diabetes, water retention, worms, systemic lupus erythematosus, tuberculosis, urinary bladder inflammation, kidney problems and externally for pain, ringworm, sprains and swellings, bruising, leech bites, eye infections, acne, inflammatory skin conditions and skin sores, soreness inside of the mouth, infected wounds, and gum disease".

It is an impressive, if slightly bizarre, list for a herb that traditionally has been limited to little more than use in digestive problems, pain relief, eye disease, urinary tract disorders, some menstrual complaints and to beautify the skin. This book attempts to cut through some of this hype, identify the real therapeutic nature of turmeric, evaluate the claims made for curcumin and the various patented extracts and make some practical suggestions for using turmeric to deliver genuine health benefits.

A note of caution

There have been cases of medicinal grade curcumin being adulterated with synthetically made substitutes, while culinary grade turmeric is often mixed with fillers – typically rice flour, chalk powder or starch – which has been coloured yellow with lead chromate or "metanil yellow", a non-permitted food colouring widely used in India which in chronic consumption can affect the nervous system[6].

It is an issue not confined to low-grade producers in parts of Asia. In 2016 Gel Spice, a US-based "importer and manufacturer of superior quality spices" was forced to recall seven different brands of ground turmeric because of high lead content – presumably from lead chromate used to colour a filler[7]. Buying from reputable sources may not be a total guarantee of quality, indeed, some Indian writers suggest only ever buying whole turmeric rhizomes. If in doubt about quality you can find methods of testing your turmeric for lead chromate and metanil yellow on the Internet[8].

In traditional Chinese medicine turmeric is contraindicated

in pregnancy and studies with rats have shown that it reduces fertility. This is not generally given as a caution on commercially available food supplements in the West, but is worth bearing in mind that only smaller culinary quantities of turmeric may be safe if you are pregnant or trying to conceive. The WHO monograph on turmeric cautions: "The safety of *Rhizoma Curcumae longae* during pregnancy has not been established. As a precautionary measure the drug should not be used during pregnancy except on medical advice"[9].

It is also worth noting a letter from two Italian researchers which appeared in *Trends in Pharmacological Sciences*, back in 2009[10]. They raised concerns about the "interaction of curcumin with drug-metabolizing enzymes and the possible repercussions in therapy" which "could be responsible for an undesired increase in plasma concentrations of drugs metabolized through these enzymes, such as digoxin, acetaminophen and morphine". In some cases, and with certain drugs, they argued that this could lead to serious and unexpected side effects, such as "the risk to develop life-threatening ventricular arrhythmias" in elderly patients prescribed amiodarone or quinidine.

If you are taking any sort of prescription medication, then it is worth discussing the potential risks of adding curcumin supplements to your diet with your doctor first.

Chapter 2

Meet the plant and its traditional uses

Turmeric (*Curcuma longa*) is a member of the ginger family – the Zingiberaceae – and is native to Southeast Asia where it grows in hot, wet, monsoon forests. It is an upright perennial reaching 1m (3ft) with long green leaves around 15–18cm (6–7in) long when fully grown and forms pale green to white petal-like leaf bracts with small yellow flower tips nestling between them when in bloom. The flowers are sterile and do not produce viable seed so the plant is propagated by rhizomes. Its rootstock is characterised by two types of small rhizomes: "primary" which are ovate or pear-shaped and are known as "bulb" or "round" turmeric and secondary, lateral rhizomes which are cylindrical and around 4–7cm long and 1–1.5cm wide known as "fingers"[1]. Other *Curcuma* species have white or blue-green rhizomes, but turmeric's are a very bright orange giving the powdered herb its distinctive shade; turmeric's "fingers" contain the most colouring material.

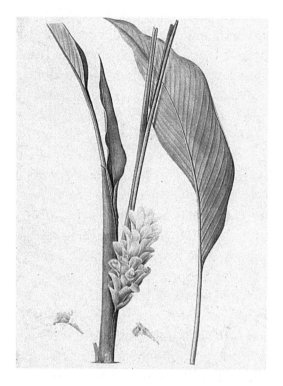

Turmeric (*Curcuma longa*) from
Pierre-Joseph Redouté (1802) *Les Lillacées*

Turmeric needs a temperature of between 20°C and 30°C (68–86°F) to grow, as well as an annual rainfall of between 1m and 2m (39–78in) – so not one for growing in a British herb garden. Typically small rhizomes are planted in the spring when the soil is warm about 30cm (12in) apart and 5cm (2in) deep. Harvesting is generally nine months later once the lower leaves of the plant have begun to wilt and turn yellow. In commercial cultivation the whole clump is generally cropped but home growers, in areas with a suitable climate, can just ease rhizomes from around the edges of the plant. After three or four years the clumps need digging up and dividing.

It is possible to grow turmeric in a pot indoors, although it does require constant warmth and plenty of water. You need a large plant pot – at least a 3 litre container – and fresh rhizomes which can generally be bought from Thai food stores. Choose a couple of rhizomes with two or three buds and plant about 5cm/2in deep in good potting compost and water well. Keep the plant warm – at least 20°C/68°F all year round – and in a sunny position. The soil must also be kept moist but well-drained throughout the year. When foliage appears use a spray to mist the leaves regularly and create a humid environment for the plant. If the temperature drops to 10°C/50°F the plant is likely to suffer. If it does die down, then dig up the rhizomes, clean off any soil, store in a cool dry place and replant when the weather is warm again.

Once harvested turmeric rhizomes are prepared in various ways. In India and Pakistan they are generally steamed or boiled – for up to 6 hours in Pakistan, less in India – to remove the raw odour and gelatinise the starch content, before being dried and crushed, while in parts of Southeast Asia, they are more likely to be used fresh. Fresh turmeric leaves are used as a herb for flavouring dishes in Malay and Indonesian cookery while in Thailand the young shoots and flower tips are boiled as a vegetable or used in omelettes[3].

Although known botanically today as *C. longa,* turmeric is sometimes listed in older texts as *C. domestica.* According to Kew, it is thought to be a hybrid that developed in ancient times in South or Southeast Asia – possibly in Vietnam, China or western India – between *Curcuma aromatica* (wild turmeric) and some other closely related species. As such it is unknown in the wild and is only available in cultivation[2]. As with all plants that have been long cultivated there are also a very large number of turmeric cultivars: at least 70 are known in India which produces around 90% or the world's supplies. These cultivars all vary slightly in their chemical composition: an analysis in 2011 found that – at that time – at least 235 compounds had been identified in turmeric rhizomes[4].

Like all plants, the substances that make up a typical turmeric rhizome vary depending on cultivar, time of harvesting, circumstances of its growth and the nature of the soil in which it grew. As with all rhizomes there are a number of sugars – arabinose (about 1%), fructose (about 10%) and glucose (about 25%) – as well as abundant starch grains (about 25%), some moisture (about 10%), fats (up to 10%), protein (about 6–7%) and traces of minerals derived from the soil. Turmeric also contains volatile oil (about 5%) made up of various aromatic chemicals including aromatic turmerone, curlone (beta-turmerone) and aromatic curcumene[5].

The constituents which have attracted the most attention, however, are the curcuminoids responsible for turmeric's distinctive colour.. The group includes curcumin, demethoxycurcumin, bisdemethoxycurcumin and cyclocurcumin; curcumin makes up about 60–70% of any curcuminoid extract while demethoxycurcumin and bisdemethoxycurcumin together account for around 30% with numerous, less abundant constituents adding to the mix.

Many sorts of *Curcuma*

There are around 130 species in the *Curcuma* genus, which grow in areas stretching from the Indian subcontinent and southern China to northern Australia, but the phytochemistry of only about 20 have been investigated to any extent. Other *Curcuma* species used medicinally in various parts of India include:

- *C. amada (amhaldi)* – camphor turmeric used as a carminative and for sprains.
- *C. angustifolia* known as wild arrowroot or narrow-leaved turmeric *(tikhur kanda)* – used for broken bones, diarrhoea and jaundice as well as boiled in milk as a restorative in debility or convalescence.
- *C. aromatica* is known as wild turmeric *(jangli haldi* in India) or *vanharidra* in classical Ayurvedic texts. It has cream-coloured rather than yellow rhizomes and is taken internally as a tonic or as a carminative for digestive problems and is also used externally for sprains, bruises, and in cosmetic preparations.
- *C. caesia*, sometimes called black turmeric *(kali haldi)*, is traditionally used in similar ways to turmeric and its rhizomes are deep bluish-black in colour.
- *C. zedoaria (kachura)*, also known as zedoary, has a pale yellow rhizome. It was once used with sappan wood *(Cesalpinia sappan)* to make a red dye and also in cosmetics[6]. It can be crushed and mixed with water to make a bath used to treat jaundice[7].

There has been significant confusion in the past over which species of *Curcuma* are used in various Chinese "drugs" but a massive study[8] over the past 20 years undertaken jointly by the Royal Botanic Gardens, Kew, and the Institute of Medicinal Plant Development, Beijing, has recently been published and has identified the precise species used. These are *C. wenyujin*, *C. phaeocaulis*, *C. kwangsiensis* and turmeric, all of which may be used as *yu jin*, traditionally a remedy for abdominal and chest pains, period pains, nose bleeds, and heart disease. In Chinese theory, all these conditions may be associated with "Blood stagnation" (see Appendix 2). For *yu jin*, the various rhizomes are steamed or boiled and dried; then softened, sliced thinly (1–2mm) and dried again.

C. *phaeocaulis*, C.*kwangsiensis* and C. *wenyujin* are also used to produce a drug known as *e zhu*, which is similarly used for pains associated with "Blood stagnation". This time the rhizomes are washed, steamed or boiled, then dried in the sun before being soaked, cut into pieces 2–4mm thick and dried again. Sometimes the whole rhizomes are boiled in rice vinegar before being cut into slices and this is called *cu er zhu*.

Turmeric traditions

Yellow-orange is a significant and sacred colour in many parts of Asia possibly because it is the colour of both the sun and gold. It is easy to imagine that turmeric – a specially cultivated hybrid or possibly a naturally occurring one that was seen as having special significance – was thus selected in early times because of its colour and its use as a dyestuff. Depending on whether the turmeric solution used is acid or alkali, the colour produced can vary from yellow to red.

In Hinduism yellow is associated with the god Vishnu, while in parts of India women still colour their cheeks yellow in the evening in tribute to Lakshmi – the goddess of wealth, health, fortune and prosperity and wife of Vishnu. Turmeric was associated with marriage rituals with turmeric water poured over the hands of bride and groom in some areas, used in paste to smear the body in others, while elsewhere sorghum grains dyed with turmeric may still be thrown over the bride and groom. Strings dyed yellow with turmeric would be draped around a bride's neck on her wedding day and also used to tie the hands of the bride and groom during the ceremony – today, more affluent families use gold chains.

Turmeric mixed with lime forms a red paste – *kumkum* – which is used to make the various forehead marks or *bindi*

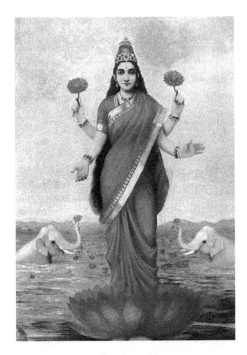

Lakshmi – Hindu goddess of wealth, fortune and prosperity,
from a painting by Ravi Varma (1896)

worn in India. In some communities newborn infants are given
turmeric and coconut milk as their first drink, while in others
turmeric water was associated with the goddess Kali and used
in sacred ablutions. In some parts of India, turmeric takes on a
sacred identity: ". . . a separate icon, known as *haridra Ganesha*
(turmeric *Ganesha*) came into existence . . . people . . . worship
Ganesha in the form of turmeric rhizome . . . Telugu people
make a cone with turmeric powder and worship it as goddess
Gowrie during the *Dasara* festival"[6].

Traditionally, turmeric was also thought to bring good luck,
and small pieces of dried rhizome were often tied to cooking
pans, carried in a pocket to prevent disease, or hung around
the neck using yellow silk thread.

In China yellow also had sacred connotations: it was the colour reserved for use by the emperor – hence all that yellow decoration in Beijing's "Forbidden City". It was also the colour associated with *Huang Di* (yellow emperor), one of the mythical founders of China who reputedly lived around 2600BC; one of China's earliest medicinal texts, the *Huang Di Nei Jing* (the Yellow Emperor's Inner Canon), takes its name from this mythical figure.

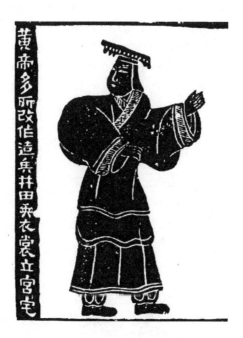

The Yellow Emperor, from a mural painting dating to the Han dynasty (206BC–220AD). Source: Li Ung Bin (1914) *Outlines of Chinese History*, Shanghai.

In Buddhism yellow and gold are the colours associated with Ratnasambhava – one of the Five Meditation Buddha's of tantric Buddhism.

As well as an important dyestuff, turmeric has also been used for millennia as a culinary spice. It has a much milder taste than other members of the Zingiberaceae (such as ginger, galangal or cardamom) with a mustard-like, earthy aroma and pungent, slightly bitter flavour. In cooking it gives colour to curries and is also used as a substitute for saffron to colour rice and other dishes, although obviously lacking saffron's distinctive flavour.

The name "turmeric" derives from the Latin *terra merita* (meritorious earth) since the ground rhizome resembles a mineral pigment. It is still known as *terre mérite* – as well as *safran des Indes* – in French. Turmeric has more than 50 names in Sanskrit, ranging from *bhadra* (lucky) to *varnini* (which gives colour) although *haridra* (dear to hari, Lord Krishna) is the most common[9].

Table 1: Some of the names for turmeric

Language	Name
Hindi	*haldi*
Sanskrit	*haridra*
Tamil	*manjal*
Thai	*khamin leung*
Indonesian	*kunyit*
Malay	*kunyit*
Philipino	*dilaw*
Mandarin	*jiang huang*
French	*terre mérite, safran des Indes*
German	*Kurkuma*
Spanish	*cúrcuma*

Turmeric as cosmetic

Turmeric has has a long history of use as a cosmetic. Women in Kerala, for example, would smear their bodies with a mixture of turmeric and sandalwood paste before bathing. This use, apparently spread to Rome, and the spice was imported in

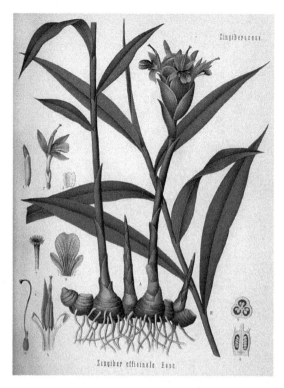

Ginger (*Zingiber officinale*) from Franz Eugen Köhler
(1897) *Köhler's Medizinal-Pflanzen*

ancient times from the Malabar Coast, and used as a beauty aid by Roman women. Turmeric water is used in India to give a golden glow to the complexion and some of the plant's ancient Sanskrit names reflect its use as a beauty aid to improve the skin: *varna-datri* – one who gives colour; *hemaragi* – golden complexion; *yoshti priya* – favourite of young women and *hridayavilasini* – giving delight to the heart.[6]

Turmeric has also long been used in parts of Asia to remove unwanted hair. Typically around half to one teaspoon of ground turmeric is mixed with a cup of gram or chickpea flour and a little milk to form a paste. This is then spread on the

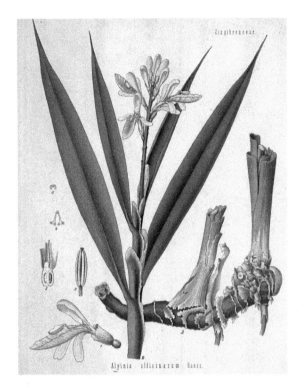

Galangal (*Alpinia officinarum*) from
Franz Eugen Köhler (1897) *Köhler's Medizinal-Pflanzen*

area to be treated, allowed to dry before being rubbed off with
a damp cloth. Yellow stains left by turmeric are traditionally
removed by rubbing with coconut oil or vinegar. Numerous
cosmetic face creams using turmeric are available in India.

Traditional Indian medicine

[See Appendix 1 for an explanation of Ayurvedic terms]

Turmeric has been regarded as a medicinal herb in Ayurvedic
tradition for at least 2,500 years. It is classified as having a

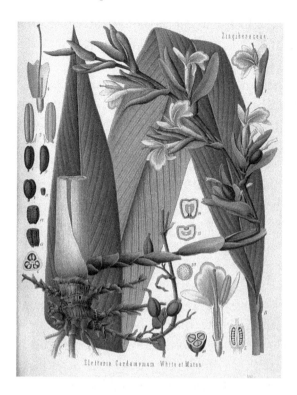

Cardamom (*Elettaria cardamomum*) from
Franz Eugen Köhler (1897) *Köhler's Medizinal-Pflanzen*

bitter and pungent taste, is *rooksha* (irritant, drying), and hot.
It is mentioned in the *Sushruta Samhita*, an ancient Ayurvedic
text generally dated to somewhere around 600BC[10]. The text
lists about 700 medicinal herbs grouped by action into numerous categories. Turmeric (*haridra*) is included in several of the
groups including:

- *Haridradi* which are "purifiers of breast milk and specifically
  act as the assimilators of the deranged humours of the body,
  their curative properties being markedly witnessed in cases of
  mucous dysentery".

- *Mustadi* which, among other attributes "cure uterine and vaginal disorders, purify the breast milk of a mother and act as good digestants".
- *Lakshadi* whose herbs have "an astringent, bitter and sweet taste and act as a good vermifuge and purifying agent in cases of bad, malignant or indolent ulcers. Diseases due to the deranged *kapha* and *pitta* prove amenable to its curative properties which extend in cases of cutaneous affections as well".
- *Vata-Samshamana-Varga* – herbs which soothe and restore *vata* to its normal state.

The *Sushruta Samhita* also includes recommended treatments for a very wide range of diseases – not all of them easily equated with our modern Western syndromes. Turmeric is suggested as a cure for several disorders, including jaundice, eye diseases, cholera, certain urinary tract problems, and some types of ulcers.

In Indian folk tradition, turmeric rhizome has been used both by itself (as a simple) or in combination with other herbs. As a simple its applications included hazy vision, eye inflammation, subnormal temperature, body pains, rheumatism, and skin sores. Well diluted in water the juice is still used in India as a cooling eyewash while more concentrated juice is used for parasitic skin infections.

Indian folk remedies using turmeric include[11]:

- boiling a teaspoon of the ground herb in milk for three minutes for coughs, sore throat or tonsillitis;
- taking a spoonful of turmeric powder in a bowl of yoghurt each morning and evening for anaemia;
- mixing half a teaspoon of turmeric with one teaspoon of aloe vera gel for cuts, wounds or fungal nail infections;
- taking a pinch of the powder twice a day for indigestion;
- mixed with ghee as an external ointment for haemorrhoids;

- while inhaling fumes of the burning rhizome was a remedy for catarrh.

Turmeric has also been used in combinations with other herbs[12]:

- with tobacco for night blindness;
- with ginger and green chickpea for scabies;
- with mustard and roots of yellow berried nightshade (*Solanum suratense*) for coughs;
- with the leaves of sweet potato, black cumin (*Nigella sativa*), and roots of *Buettneria herbacea* (a type of mallow known as *deku sindur*) to encourage lactation; or
- mixed with an equal amount of red sandalwood powder and distilled water as a paste for styes.

Turmeric flowers have been used for throat sores, indigestion, cholera, and syphilis – in this case combined with the flowers of *Shorea robusta* (sal or shala tree) and the bark of *Ventilago calyculata* (a type of vine or liana)[12].

Modern Ayurvedic practitioners take a broader approach to turmeric's properties. One herbal[13] suggests it can be used for indigestion, poor circulation, coughs, pharyngitis, skin disorders, diabetes, arthritis, anaemia, wounds, bruises, an absence of menstrual periods and describes it as "an excellent natural antibiotic ... [it] strengthens digestion and helps improve menstrual flora".

Traditional Chinese medicine

[See Appendix 2 for an explanation of Chinese medical terms]

Turmeric is not a native of China although it is now cultivated there. Although it can sometimes be used as one of the herbs that can be called *yu jin*, it is more likely to be found as *jiang huang* – a name that translates as "ginger yellow".

The herb is first mentioned in the *Tang Materia Medica* which dates from around 659AD[14] and is defined as "pungent, bitter and warm"– although some Chinese herbalists regard it as cool rather than warm. In Chinese theory it is said to "invigorate the Blood" so it can be used for both pain associated with "Blood stagnation" and menstrual disorders, including period pain and an absence of menstruation. As an invigorating herb it is also said to "move *qi*". Like "Blood stagnation", "stagnant *qi*" is seen in Chinese theory as a cause of pain. Turmeric is used for various types of abdominal pain and to "expel wind" – regarded as another cause of painful conditions, especially pain in the shoulders. Turmeric is also said to "scatter constraint, strengthen the function of the Heart and Spleen and repel epidemic disease"[15].

As a herb which can clear Blood stagnation, *jiang huang* is contraindicated in pregnancy, since in classic Chinese theory the pregnant uterus and foetus qualify as an aspect of stagnant Blood. It is a significant caution as in the West turmeric is often regarded as quite safe to use in pregnancy, although its traditional use in promoting menstruation should ring alarm bells.

Although most Chinese herbs are used in complex combinations, turmeric is more often prescribed as a single herb and the ground powder is known as *jiang huang san*. It is also used in some standard formulations. *Sheng jiang san*, for example, contains ten herbal ingredients apart from turmeric and is also known as "ascending and descending powder" and is used to treat a wide range of ailments associated with Liver heat and disordered *qi*[16]. *Jin gu die da wan* includes an even longer list of herbs and is used to clear Blood stagnation and speed recovery from injury: the mixture is sometimes sold as "bruise mender".

Western herbal approaches to turmeric

Turmeric is a comparative newcomer to the western herbal tradition. Writing in 1930, Maud Grieve[17] gives it scant attention describing it as "a mild aromatic stimulant seldom used in medicine except as a colouring. It was once a cure for jaundice". She adds that it is "chiefly used" in curry powder, "as an adulterant of mustard ... and one of the ingredients of many cattle condiments".

Research into turmeric in recent decades has begun to change this view, although herbals initially recommended a comparatively narrow range of ailments where it could be helpful. By 2000 applications listed in Mills and Bone's seminal textbook[18] for either turmeric or its curcumin extract "supported by clinical trials" included rheumatoid arthritis, osteoarthritis, and indigestion, with "traditional uses" given as topically for skin disorders and internally for poor digestion and liver function.[18]

By the 2013 second edition of this book[19] its lists were significantly expanded: the range of ailments for curcumin "supported by clinical trials" now included "postoperative inflammation, precancerous conditions, tropical pancreatitis (with piperine), induction of gallbladder contraction, stabilisation of inflammatory bowel disease, HIV-associated chronic diarrhoea, chronic anterior uveitis, psoriasis, and monoclonal gammopathy".

Most had the additional proviso that the trial had been "uncontrolled" – i.e. the results were not compared with a control group of sufferers taking placebo so there is no measure of the "placebo effect" which is where sufferers report an improvement due to the very fact of being given "new" medication by doctors who are taking an interest in their condition. Additional applications for turmeric listed by Bone and Mills were: "elevated blood lipids, precancerous lesions, and irritable bowel syndrome" – again all based on uncontrolled trials[19].

Herbals generally also give a list of actions for plants. These are often based on animal studies or *in vitro* tests. Adding a chemical to a colony of bacteria in a petri dish or cells in a test tube (*in vitro*) is very different from oral ingestion by real people, due to the fact that chemicals may break down in the digestive process or simply be excreted unchanged and unabsorbed – a particular problem with curcumin, as discussed in the next chapter.

As with lists of ailments, actions claimed for turmeric have steadily multiplied over the years. The 1988 revised edition of *Potter's Cyclopaedia*[20] followed Mrs Grieve in pointing out that turmeric is "seldom used medicinally", adding that "recent research has shown many useful properties . . . particularly the anti-inflammatory and anti-hepatoxic effects" and included the results of some 1980s trials such as demonstrating that turmeric "has anti-fertility effects in rats" and is "antibiotic *in vitro*".

By 1995, Thomas Bartram[21] listed turmeric as "aromatic, blood purifier, anti-oxidant, carminative, cholagogue, choleretic, bile stimulant, detoxifier, regenerator for liver tissue; anti-inflammatory for arthritis, skin disorders and asthma; anti-tumour activity, anti-cancer".

Five years later in their 2000 edition, Mills and Bone list:[18] anti-inflammatory, anti-platelet, anti-oxidant, hypolipidaemic, choleretic, anti-microbial, carminative, depurative" but by the the 2013 edition[19] the list had grown to: "anti-inflammatory, anti-oxidant, hypolipidaemic, choleretic, cholagogue, anti-microbial, carminative, depurative, anti-carcinogenic, anti-tumour, radioprotective, neuroprotective, hepatoprotective, nephroprotective, cardioprotective, vasoprotective."

To say there is some confusion as to what exactly turmeric does would appear to be an understatement.

Chapter 3

Focussing on the curcuminoids

Curcumin – or diferuloyl methane to give it one of its scientific names – is a hydrophobic polyphenol with a lengthy list of attributed pharmacological activities. The Curcumin Resource Database (CRDB)[1] identifies 176 different turmeric cultivars with measured curcumin content for each varying from just over 1% to one or two plants that provide as much as 10%[1].

Hydrophobic indicates that the chemical is not soluble in water. Curcumin will dissolve in boiling water but precipitates out again when the water cools. Instead it is fat soluble – which is exactly the same as vitamins A, D, E and K. Polyphenols are naturally occurring chemicals in plants which, among other things, are involved in the release of the plant's growth hormones, help to protect it from ultra-violet radiation, prevent microbial infections and deter herbivores. Soluble polyphenols are among the constituents frequently found in herbal teas and are often regarded as key constituents contributing to a herb's therapeutic properties.

Curcumin was first extracted from turmeric back in 1815[2] by stirring the powder for several hours in a suitable solvent to dissolve the hydrophobic part, which was then collected by filtration and evaporation of the solvent. Various solvents have been used for extraction over the years including ethanol, hexane, and acetone as well as food grade triacylglycerols. Once extracted the solvent is evaporated and the residue cleaned. Curcumin can also be extracted using supercritical carbon dioxide as solvent (at above 31°C and a pressure of above 74bar) which avoids leaving residues on the extracted material as the carbon dioxide turns back to gas when at normal pressure. This process is widely used to produce such foods as decaffeinated coffee.

However the extraction is performed, the result is a mixture of chemicals which can be further separated by using high performance liquid chromatography (HPLC) or column chromatography. The curcumin segment can then be identified and isolated. Solvents – such as methanol and chloroform – are needed again at this stage to provide a suitable medium for the chromatography machine so the final extract needs further cleansing to remove any traces that remain.

More recently new techniques to improve the water solubility of curcumin have been introduced, including attaching the curcumin molecule to nanoparticles of silicon or metal oxides. The technique is already used in the pharmaceutical industry to improve the water solubility of certain drugs. Inevitably introducing another substance into the curcumin extract could change its therapeutic properties and some recent research has focussed on identifying how these new nanocomposites perform[3].

Curcumin was first synthesised in 1928. It is not an especially complex process and there have been several cases in recent years of curcumin "extracts" adulterated with the synthetic chemical, which can be identified using radiocarbon testing. In 2015, for example, Indian police impounded curcumin products made by Bayir Extracts which contained up to 45% synthetic material[4].

Synthetically produced curcumin is not the only adulterant that has been found in turmeric or curcumin food supplements. In 2009 the Medicines and Healthcare Products Regulatory Agency (MHRA) issued a warning about a turmeric-based food supplement called Fortodol (also sold as Miradin). This had been found to contain a strong anti-inflammatory drug called nimesulide which can cause serious damage to the liver and is not licensed as a medicine in the UK. The product was recalled, but not before it had been linked to serious liver problems (including one fatality) involving 11 patients in Sweden and five in Norway[5].

Chemical extras

In theory, synthetic curcumin should behave exactly as naturally-extracted curcumin, but that natural curcumin is not always quite what it seems. Most extracts – even some which claim to be refined – are, as discussed earlier, a mixture of closely related compounds, the curcuminoids (including demethoxycurcumin, bisdemethoxycurcumin and cyclocurcumin) plus small quantities of other chemicals. All these chemicals are classed as "secondary metabolites" – organic compounds that are not directly involved in the normal growth, development, or reproduction of the plant. The structure of the curcumin molecule also changes depending on the acidity of the medium in which it happens to be found. The more alkaline its surroundings, the more likely curcumin will add an extra hydrogen atom and take what is called the "keto" form, otherwise it exists in what the chemists call an "enol" form – flipping between structures like this is called tautomerism. Curcumin also breaks down on exposure to sunlight and in various water and water-organic solutions, producing a new clutch of degradation substances such as ferulic acid and vanillin (from which it is often synthesised) adding to the mix.

Chemical structures of curcumin tautomers

So natural "curcumin" – extracted using solvents at some stage in the process – is "multicomponent": a mixture of several different compounds which will vary depending on the extraction process and the degree of light the mixture has been exposed to. Interestingly, the 2017 review led by Michael Walters, a medicinal chemist at the University of Minnesota[6], notes that many of the research studies *"in vitro"* used pure, synthetic curcumin, while *"in vivo"* studies and clinical trials tended to use natural extracts, i.e. a "curcuminoid" mixture. As cases of adulteration of "natural" curcumin with the synthetically produced chemical are known, it is difficult to see how these various studies can all be regarded as involving the same, identical substance.

Chemical structure of demethoxycurcumin

Chemical structure of bisdemethoxycurcumin

Walters' review details at length the various problems associated with any curcumin trial since the actual material used
is effectively an unknown mixture comprising "... the assumed
bioactive material *and any impurities*" (their italics) at all times.
In addition the typical time frame for any of these studies
means that any curcumin present will start to degrade, so there
will be an unknown assortment of degradation products in the
mix that will vary over time. This – and other factors relating
to the instability of the curcumin molecule in solution – mean
that studies often prove difficult to replicate and clinical trials
do not always give consistent results.

Speaking to the scientific publication *Nature*, Michael
Walters described the focus on curcumin as "a cautionary
tale"[7], while editor in chief of the journal which published the
review, Gunda Georg, declared that "much effort and funding
has been wasted on curcumin research".

Chemical structure of cyclocurcumin

The scientists involved in Walters' extensive review have all "declared no competing financial interest" and only one lists any previous employment with pharmaceutical companies, so they can be excused of bias against a herbal product. Similarly, no pharmaceutical companies were involved in funding the study. The review team concluded that there was "much ado about nothing" with respect to the *in vivo* studies and clinical trials using curcumin or curcuminoid extracts, although they "do not rule out that an extract of crude turmeric might have beneficial effects on human health".

What is questionable, however, is whether or not curcumin really is the only significant constituent of turmeric and should it be credited with the growing range of attributes claimed for it?

In vitro studies may be relevant if the curcumin is to be used topically and thus bypass the digestive tract, but are of little use in predicting how curcumin will behave when taken orally since it either breaks down during the digestive process or ends up being flushed down the lavatory pan unchanged, having never even entered the blood stream. One early study in the 1970s involving rats found that 75% of orally ingested curcumin passed through the rats' digestive tracts unchanged and was found in their faeces. Negligible amounts were found in urine and injected curcumin was metabolised within 30 minutes. The authors concluded: "In view of the poor absorption, rapid metabolism and excretion of curcumin, it is unlikely that substantial concentrations of curcumin occur in the body after ingestion"[8].

Various curcumin "phase-2" metabolites – substances produced during the digestion process – have also been identified[9]. Investigations have been limited but one of these breakdown products, tetrahydrocurcumin[10], demonstrated chemopreventative [i.e. anti-cancer] properties in rats, so possibly these breakdown products have some therapeutic activity that has yet to be fully explored.

While turmeric has a distinctive bright yellow colour, attributed to the curcuminoids, it is not the only member of the genus to contain these chemicals. A study[11] looking at the constituents of several *Curcuma* species found that zedoary (*C. zeodaria*) and wild arrowroot (*C. angustifolia*) also contained significant amounts of curcumin (see Table 2) and these species also share some of the traditional therapeutic uses of turmeric.

Table 2: Content of total curcumin in six different species of Curcuma[11]

Name of plant species	Curcumin content mg/100g
C. amada	11
C. angustifolia	71
C. caesia	8
C. leucorrhiza	15
C. longa	125
C. zedoaria	88

It leaves numerous question marks over whether curcumin, the wider group of curcuminoids or the phase-2 metabolites, produced during the digestive process, are responsible for any perceived therapeutic effects of curcumin extracts.

Despite the preoccupation with curcumin, other studies have focussed on the components of turmeric's volatile oil and have demonstrated that some of these – the turmerones – display potent anti-fungal and anti-bacterial activity and are thus being studied by some researchers as a source of new antibiotics[12]. So is it better to look for a remedy containing turmerones if the health problem involves an infection?

Patenting the extracts

Once curcumin had been identified and synthesised, the next stage for the scientists and manufacturers was to investigate its potential therapeutic attributes with a view to developing a patentable drug. The earliest scientific paper on the CRDB (Curcumin Research DataBase) dates from 1919, with the next – a study of curcumin in treating biliary disease – dated 1937, followed by a third on anti-bacterial properties of curcumin in 1949. After that the publishing pace grew steadily reaching those 1,400 papers involving curcumin that appeared in 2016. By the 1990s numerous manufacturers were patenting curcumin extracts for a range of applications – from its use as a dyestuff, to remedies containing curcumin for treating skin problems in pets, to different extraction methods for obtaining curcuminoid mixtures.

Today, there are several companies producing patented curcuminoid extracts which are then used by the food supplement producers to make consumer products. These patented extracts are generally identified in the small print of the label on the capsule tub and most have been treated in some way to improve water solubility and absorption

A challenge for the makers of extracts has been to produce a type of curcumin that will be absorbed by the body and their promotional material generally focusses on "bioavailability" – i.e. how much of the curcumin present will actually be absorbed into the blood stream and remain there for long enough to have a therapeutic effect. Curcumin content and its bioavailability are seen as key differentiators between the various products with numerous Internet blogs, Youtube videos, and marketing campaigns attempting to highlight the advantages of extract X over extract Y. However, given its hydrophobic nature and tendency to degrade it seems likely that bioavailability must vary over time depending on the age of the final consumer product, the conditions in which it is stored and so on.

The earliest curcumin extracts were simply the curcuminoid portion from the chromatography machine which had been further refined to increase the proportion of curcumin. As concerns over bioavailability increased, some producers started to recommend the addition of black pepper – known to increase the bioavailability of other fat soluble drugs. Since the 1990s, new curcumin extracts have continued to appear, each claiming to increase bioavailability significantly, while almost all the marketing messages, and much of the associated research by companies producing curcumin extracts, continues to be based on the premise that curcumin alone is responsible for turmeric's therapeutic properties.

A few do take a different approach. BCM-95® (see p.39), for example, stresses that its product also contains an extract from turmeric's essential oil, while one study using the curcumin extract Meriva®[13] noted that: "... the major plasma curcuminoid after administration of Meriva was not curcumin, but demethoxycurcumin [one of the curcuminoids] a more potent analogue in many *in vitro* anti-inflammatory assays"[14].

Statements such as this add to the confusion. If demethoxycurcumin is more potent that curcumin in some tests, then why do the producers of curcumin extracts cast aspersions on their rivals who sell products with a higher concentration of the other curcuminoids?

The manufacturers of each of these various extracts sponsor clinical trials using their particular product, so it can be difficult to compare the efficacy of the various patented extracts as there are very few clinical trials that involve or compare several. Equally, it is possible that these companies will only encourage publication of research which shows their products in a beneficial light. All producers list details of their sponsored – and always successful – tests and clinical trials on their websites. Many of these are *in vitro* studies while clinical trials often involve very few patients and may be uncontrolled, thus making the significance of any results – given the placebo effect – potentially questionable. Many trials conclude that further studies are needed.

Extract producers also claim that their particular product will increase bioavailability by anything from "20-fold" to ". . . 285 times" that of "standard 95% curcumin". If, as those early studies on rats suggested, bioavailability of curcumin beyond the gastro-intestinal tract is minimal, then 285 times not a lot doesn't add up to very much.

Chapter 4

Extracts and supplements

At the time of writing, the Curcuma Research DataBase, lists 962 different patents for curcumin. Many of the most recent relate to formatting curcumin as nanoparticles or creating more soluble forms on the chemical by various means. Several are from companies which already produce commercial curcumin extracts, but some are from other extract producers clearly interested in entering the field – so we can probably expect more branded curcumin extracts, claiming even greater bioavailability to appear in future[1].

Some of the currently available branded extracts are:

Curcumin C3 Complex®

This is a "≥95% curcumin standardised turmeric extract" produced and patented by Sabinsa Corporation based in the USA. Sabinsa's first patent for the extract was issued in 1999 making it one of the older curcumin extracts currently used by food supplement

manufacturers. It contains the three major curcuminoids (i.e. curcumin, demethoxycurcumin and bisdemethoxycurcumin) which,
they say account for 95% or more of its extract.

Sabinsa also manufactures BioPerine®, which is a piperine
extract from black pepper. It increases the bioavailability of
various vitamins and minerals, such as selenium and vitamin
C, as well as curcumin. Research in 1997[2] found that piperine
increased the bioavailability of curcumin by 20-fold "... in
both rats and humans with no adverse effects". A more recent
study[3] concluded: "Co-administration of piperine significantly
enhanced the effect of curcumin (25mg/kg) but not of curcumin (50mg/kg)". A dose of 25mg/kg works out at about 1.6g
for a person weighing 10 stones (63kg).

Unlike some of the other primary manufacturers, Sabinsa
lists the companies which use Curcumin C3 Complex® in
consumer products on its website. Currently 21 are cited and
Sabinsa adds: "As and when we identify more customers who
are using Curcumin C3 Complex®, we will report that here".
The products vary significantly: some contain 250mg "turmeric
root standardised to contain 95% curcuminoids" others 500mg
or even 1100mg.

According to some commentators[4] "... curcumin 95% with
piperine is most often used because it was one of the first
curcumin extracts available for manufacturers ... and it is
inexpensive". Certainly it does seem to appear more frequently
on the health food store shelves than many other extracts.

http://www.sabinsa.com
http://www.curcuminoids.com

Longvida®

Longvida® is produced by Verdure Sciences in the USA. The
company describes it as "Optimized Curcumin ... optimized

to deliver free curcumin into target tissues through the critical bioavailability requirements of permeability, solubility, and stability". It also claims that Longvida® is "... at least 67–285 times more bioavailable than standard 95% curcumin". The product was patented in 2006 and has been used in numerous clinical trials since at least 2009.

Longvida is a "solid lipid particle formulation" comprising 20% curcumin and 80% phospholipids, which provide the curcumin particles with a non-aqueous medium in which to dissolve. This is said to speed absorption of the curcumin into the blood stream and it can cross the blood-brain barrier. As a result Longvida® research has tended to focus on its use in treating brain-related conditions including Alzheimer's disease and traumatic brain injuries. One study[5] suggests that within an hour of taking a single dose of the extract it "... significantly improved performance on sustained attention and working memory tasks, compared with placebo" for a group of healthy 60–65 year old adults.

Typical supplements contain 400–500mg of the Longvida® preparation of which 20% will be curcumin.

http://www.longvida.com

http://vs-corp.com/ingredients/longvida/

Meriva®

Meriva® is produced by Indena SpA, an Italian company based in Milan, specialising in making plant extracts. Its curcumin extract was patented in 2006 and, like Longvida® it uses phospholipids (in this case phosphatidylcholine from soya) to create an extract which is composed of between around 18% and 22% curcuminoids within the phospholipid mix.

A bioavailability study in 2011[6] involving nine people comparing Meriva® with a standard curcuminoid mixture found that: "Total curcuminoid absorption was about 29-fold higher for Meriva® than for its corresponding unformulated curcuminoid mixture, but only phase-2 metabolites could be detected, and plasma concentrations were still significantly lower than those required for the inhibition of most anti-inflammatory targets of curcumin". In other words, all the curcumin was broken down in the digestive process. However, it also found that the "phospholipid formulation increased the absorption of demethoxylated curcuminoids much more than that of curcumin, with significant differences in plasma curcuminoid profile between Meriva® and its corresponding unformulated curcuminoid mixture. Thus, the major plasma curcuminoid after administration of Meriva was not curcumin, but demethoxycurcumin, a more potent analogue in many *in vitro* anti-inflammatory assays".

Research by Indena (sometimes also involving Usana Health Sciences, a US producer of various nutritional products which uses Meriva® in some of them) has involved more than 22 clinical trials which have included its use in cancer, sports injuries, eye inflammations, neurological disorders, pain relief, diabetes, liver disorders and osteoarthritis. Some sources suggest that because of its curcuminoid mix and the increased plasma levels of demethoxycurcumin it can provide, it can be more effective that other types of extracts at suppressing inflammation.

Typical capsules using Meriva® provide between 250mg and 500mg of the preparation, so around 20% curcuminoids.

http://www.indena.com/products/meriva-personal-care/

Theracurmin®

Theracurmin® is produced by Japanese company, Theravalues Corporation. It also aims to improve the solubility of curcumin and is described as using "... fine granulation and suspension

technology, Theracurmin® is in the form of sub-micron particles that are stabilised when dispersed in water". The product
was patented in 2009 and is a mixture of curcuminoids which
have been very finely ground (to 1μm or less) in a colloidal
suspension with glycerin and a vegetable gum called gum
ghatti [mainly consisting of polysaccharides from the sap of
ghatti trees (*Anogeissus latifolia*)] which can then be more easily
absorbed into the blood.

Theravalues claims that its Theracurmin® is 27 times more
bioavailable that "ordinary curcumin powder" and that the
extract has high stability when dispersed in water and when
exposed to light, all due to the stabilising nature of its colloidal
base. The company highlights research using the extract which
demonstrates it performs better than placebo in small clinical
trials involving liver function, muscle stiffness, heart failure,
knee osteoarthritis and skin ageing, amongst other conditions[7].

Typical 300mg capsules using the extract contain 30%
curcumin (90mg)[8].

http://theravalues.com/english/

BCM-95®

BCM-95®, also sometimes called BioCurMax-95, was patented
in 2006 and is a registered trademark of USA-based DolCas
Biotech while the extract is supplied by Arjuna Natural
Extracts, an Indian company based in Kerala. The product
combines 86% curcuminoids with extracts from turmeric oil
including aromatic-turmerone, which is found in both turmeric
and mango ginger (*C. amada*), with smaller amounts of curlone (beta-turmerone) and alpha-turmerone. The extract was
patented by Arjuna in 2006. It is described by the company
as "lipophilic" – fat loving – so, as with Longvida®, it helps
to provide a suitable fat soluble medium for curcumin which

can improve absorption. BCM-95® is said to provide "7-times bioavailability of standard curcumin powder". Like other producers Arjuna details a raft of scientific reports involving BCM-95® – some *in vitro* studies, some clinical trials. It claims that the extract is indicated for: "inflammatory conditions, metabolic disorders, rheumatoid and osteoarthritis, depression, Alzheimer's and other neurological diseases, liver disease, and gastric disorders".

Essential oils are sometimes described as herbal medicine's "magic bullets" so although the turmerone content of BCM-95® may be there to improve bioavailability, it also has therapeutic properties of its own. Turmeric's essential oil comprises up to 30% of aromatic-turmerone which, according to one review[9] "... is a mosquito repellent and may be an effective drug for the treatment of respiratory disease and dermatophytosis [i.e. fungal skin infections such as ringworm]". As well as demonstrating anti-fungal and anti-bacterial properties, synthetic turmerone is said to be anti-carcinogenic, while turmeric oil also contains beta-elemene which has also demonstrated some anti-carcinogenic properties, although trials are inconclusive. It is thus uncertain what the turmeric oil may be adding to the properties of BCM-95®, but it clearly adds something,

One recent study[10] detailed by DolCas Biotech involved 110 subjects suffering from "major depressive disorder" and used doses of 500mg of BCM-95® combined with 30mg of saffron or 1000mg of BCM-95® per day both compared with placebo. Both groups taking the curcumin medication showed similar improvement in symptoms over a 12-week study compared with placebo, although the placebo group also improved during the first four weeks of the study – a common response in many trials that is generally attributed to the placebo effect and often makes accurate interpretation of any results challenging. The researchers in this study admit that: "Investigations with larger sample sizes are required to examine the efficacy of differing doses of curcumin and saffron/curcumin combination".

BCM-95® capsules on the market contain between 400mg and 750mg of which 86% (between about 340 and 640mg) comprises the curcuminoid mixture.

http://www.arjunanatural.com/bcm95.html
http://dolcas-biotech.com/products/bcm95/

NovaSOL®Curcumin

NovaSOL® products are developed by Aquanova AG in Germany. The brand is used for a range of liquid solutions ("solubilisates") which, rather like the Theravalues product, are actually colloids; here the particles are so "ultrafine" that they are smaller than the wavelength of light so the liquid appears to be a clear solution. Aquanova says that its solubilisates are both water and fat soluble (ambiphilates), are extremely stable and deliver high bioavailability. These clear liquids are then supplied to manufacturing partners who turn them into capsules or other products.

NovoSOL®Curcumin, introduced in 2013, for example, is supplied to Molecular Health Technologies in the USA which produces the curcumin capsules used in remedies such as "Solgar Full Spectrum Curcumin". It is claimed that NovoSOL®Curcumin offers "185-times" the bioavailability of pure standard curcumin. Its literature argues that "most curcumin is excreted out through the liver within 2 hours of ingesting and NovaSOL® curcumin remains in the plasma for over 24 hours!".

A typical 800mg capsule will provide 48mg of curcuminoids.
http://www.aquanova.de
http://molecularhealthtech.com
http://novasolcurcumin.com

Ateronon ACTIVE (now Turmeric+)

This was launched in 2015 by Cambridge Nutraceuticals, a UK company which claims it is "30-times more absorbable that dietary turmeric". An early study involved Spain's national Olympic Training Centre in Barcelona where doctors used Turmeric+ to treat muscle injuries. This curcumin extract is bound with a phospholipid made from soy lecithin, and the company argues that this prevents degradation of curcumin in the stomach where normally "99.8% disintegrates", so that the curcumin can then pass into the intestine where it is absorbed into the blood stream. Given its comparatively recent launch there appears to be little published information, as yet, about its use in any clinical trials – although the Spanish Olympians were so enthusiastic that the extract is now also used by Barcelona FC and, says Cambridge Nutraceuticals, "doctors and physios working at Athletico Bilbao".

http://camnutra.com

CurcuWIN®

CurcuWIN® is produced by OmniActive, which is headquartered in Mumbai while its global sales and marketing operation is based in New Jersey. OmniActive uses its "UltraSOL Nutrient Delivery System" for the extract. This is described as converting "lipophilic compounds and poorly absorbed nutrients to water dispersible ingredients for enhanced bio-availability". It mixes curcumin with an anti-oxidant (such as vitamin E), a hydrophilic carrier (believed in this case to be polyvinylpyrrolidone) and a fat in a solvent[11] which is then heated to evaporate the solvent and form a "dry mass". This is then ground into a fine powder. Polyvinylpyrrolidone is used as a binder in many pharmaceutical drugs and beauty products. CurcuWIN® contains 20% curcuminoids in the same proportions as found in natural turmeric.

In a comparison with two other curcumin extracts "a curcumin phytosome formulation" and "a formulation with volatile oils of turmeric rhizome" – believed to be Meriva® and BCM-9® – a study sponsored by OmniActive[12] demonstrated that it increased bioavailability by 46-times compared with "unformulated standard curcumin". The "formulation with volatile oils of turmeric rhizome" came second, increasing bioavailability by 35-times. The study involved "12 healthy volunteers" consuming the equivalent of 376mg of curcuminoids.

The initial patent for the manufacturing process dates from 2012 while the company obtained a US patent in September 2017 specifying that the extract is for "improving muscle performance, endurance capacity and resistance to fatigue when administered in effective amounts in humans undergoing exercise"[13]. This patent, claims the company, "addresses the needs of a much broader population including those who are living active lifestyles" – which moves a curcumin product from focussing on easing specific ailments to becoming a general supplement for the "needs of a modern, active lifestyle further expanding on curcumin's potential".

Typical supplements containing CurcuWIN® contain between 250mg and 500mg and deliver 50–100mg of curcuminoids.

http://omniactives.com/curcuwin

MetaCurcumin

MetaCurcumin is a liquid curcumin extract produced by RevGenetics, a Florida-based company which manufacturers longevity supplements and describes its product as for "inflammaging". It appears to contain nanoparticles of curcumin within a hydrophilic micelle which, it claims increases absorption "277-times". Its claims are sourced to "manufacturers, studies & product labels" but it gives no other references for them. The extract is available in a liquid pump or capsules which claim to provide 120mg of curcuminoids.

http://www.revgenetics.com

Cavacurmin®

Cavacurmin is produced by Wacker Chemie AG – a German-based global chemical company whose interests range from polymers and construction to electrical systems and healthcare. It is a comparatively new product which is not yet widely available commercially. It is produced by basically inserting the hydrophobic curcumin inside a doughnut of gamma-cyclodextrin (a type of sugar made from starch) so giving a hydrophilic exterior, which can then be absorbed. An initial study, published in February 2017, suggests bioavailability of 40-times standard curcumin[14]. As with the CurcuWIN research, this compared the bioavailability of Cavacurmin with other curcumin extracts (again probably Meriva® and BCM-95® as well as standardised 95% curcumin)

https://www.wacker.com/cms/en/industries/food/curcumin.jsp

Turmipure™

Turmipure™ was launched by French botanical products specialist Naturex[15] in June 2017. Rather than stressing bioavailability it focusses on sustainability and traceability, sourcing its organic turmeric from South India. It describes the product as "standardised up to 95% curcuminoids" and currently only promotes it for "joint health". As yet the company provides no data on bioavailability or clinical trials.

http://www.naturex.com

In addition to these branded and patented curcumin extracts, there are dozens of companies – many of them in China or India – offering various grades of powdered turmeric and curcumin extracts, including 95–99% curcumin, priced from US$10 to US$250 per kilogram. It is possible that the "food grade" varieties of these many extracts may well end up in some over-the-counter curcumin capsules[16].

Dosages

Given the variation in claimed bioavailability it is difficult to compare recommended dosages of the various curcumin/curcuminoid extracts with any degree of accuracy. Many of the food supplement producers that buy these extracts also use them in combination with other ingredients to produce differentiated remedies. It can make choosing an appropriate turmeric remedy to treat a specific complaint extremely challenging for consumers.

According to the European Food Safety Authority the acceptable daily consumption for curcumin in food products, where it is used as a colorant, is 3mg/kg bodyweight[17] so around 190mg for a 10st (63kg) individual. Research studies that appear to produce a therapeutic effect tend to administer anything from 500mg curcuminoids to 7.5g daily – even 12g a day is not unknown.

One product containing "95% curcuminoid extract", for example, gives the product break down for one 500mg capsule as containing "350mg of 95% curcuminoid powder, 150mg of powdered turmeric root and 3mg of BioPerine® black pepper extract". Dosages of up to 1500mg daily are recommended for this product "for general anti-oxidant and wellbeing and more serious anti-inflammatory disorders such as rheumatoid arthritis and other more serious ailments (diabetes, inflammatory bowel disease etc)". The producer also advises customers to "try taking whole peppercorns (2 or 3) with your supplement" if users feel the curcumin is not having as much effect as it should. Turmeric typically contains around 4.5% of curcuminoids so this particular product would appear to deliver about 340mg of curcuminoids per capsule or about 1g daily on the maximum recommended daily dose.

In contrast 500mg Longvida® capsules would have about 100mg of curcumin, while Meriva® – "18–22% curcuminoids" – would have a similar amount of curcuminoids, perhaps 90–110mg curcumin. Dosages for both are typically one or two capsules daily. NovaSOL capsules – claiming 185-times bioavailability – are at the lower end of the dosage level, typically containing 48mg of curcuminoids of which around 40mg are said to be curcumin. All these amounts are well below the quantities generally used in clinical trials and while some simply contain the patented curcumin or curcuminoid extract, other brands of capsules add ground turmeric powder. Whether this is to reduce the production cost per capsule or because of perceived benefit of bulking out the curcumin with the rest of the turmeric rhizome is hard to tell.

Capsules containing only powdered turmeric are widely available and typically will have a dose of 2 × 400mg capsules per day. A 400mg capsule would contain about (average 4.5%) 18mg of curcuminoids of which perhaps 12mg will be curcumin – so about 24mg in the daily dose. As discussed earlier, a typical recommended dose of turmeric by a medical herbalist today would contain about 360–450mg of curcumin daily – rather more than contained in many over-the-counter curcumin preparations.

Given the doubts raised over whether curcumin really is the key active constituent in turmeric, some consumers may prefer to use a product based on ground turmeric powder, or to hedge their bets by using a curcuminoid and turmeric mixture – or simply stir a spoonful of turmeric powder into their daily porridge, rice or mashed potatoes.

All sorts of supplements

While much emphasis is on patented curcuminoid extracts, some food supplement producers prefer to differentiate their products by adding additional herbs, vitamins or other assorted active ingredients. These various formulations generally give very little specific evidence of their efficacy. Supporting studies, if any, tend to be based on *in vitro* experiments of the individual herbs (or their constituents) used in the mix as well as basic facts about any vitamins added rather than any clinical trials involving the complete formulations. They may also sometimes refer to clinical trials undertaken by the various extract manufacturers involved. As all medical herbalists are well aware, herbs interact together in ways which are poorly researched and little understood and many of the combinations on offer may be delivering additional – and unknown – therapeutic benefits or otherwise.

Several supplement producers, for example, combine curcuminoids with other anti-inflammatory herbs when promoting remedies for joint problems, so it is difficult to know whether the turmeric extract is the most effective ingredient, or if any therapeutic effect is due to the added extras or maybe it is the combination acting in synergy. One BCM-95® product, for example, promoted as an anti-inflammatory, adds ginger and *Boswellia serrata* (one of the plants that produces frankincense in this case "Indian frankincense" or *shallaki*) to its capsules.

Indian frankincense is a traditional Ayurvedic remedy for arthritis, which is currently regarded as a potential alternative to non-steroidal anti-inflammatory drugs (NSAIDs)[18]. This particular supplement contains 240g each of BCM-95® and turmeric powder as well as 50mg of "ginger extract" and 100mg of the *Boswellia*. This would give a combined curcuminoid yield of around 215mg of which around 150mg may be curcumin, as well as about 25mg of the turmerones.

Another producer promoting a remedy for "joint and inflammation support" combines turmeric root (375mg) – not curcumin in this case – with 300mg *Boswellia serrata* extract and 2.5mg of BioPerine® (black pepper extract). As whole turmeric root powder is used here, the likely curcuminoid content per capsule would be around 18mg.

Some of the many other assorted supplements based on curcumin include:

- NovaSol®Curcumin (713mg) with ginger extract, vitamin C and vitamin D3 to provide "targeted support for joints, inflammation and the immune system too";
- curcumin combined with artichoke leaf extract and promoted as a digestive supplement;
- curcumin with vitamin D for reasons which the product's promotional material doesn't make entirely clear, although having expounded the importance of vitamin D in their literature, they add "curcumin is an extremely popular and media trending ingredient";
- 50mg of Curcumin C3® with 520mg ginger, 75mg tomato, 500IU vitamin D and 2.5mg BioPerine® as a "daily supplement" to help the immune system, muscle function, cell division, "blood calcium concentrations" and "normal bone and teeth";
- turmeric (300mg) with Peruvian cat's claw (100mg) and

gotu kola (100mg). Peruvian cat's claw (*Uncaria tomentosa*) is traditionally used to treat digestive problems, asthma, liver disease and arthritis – as well as being used as a contraceptive by some South American tribes. Gotu kola (*Centella asiatica*) is an important Ayurvedic rejuvenative tonic also used for skin disorders, nervous problems, and as a laxative and blood cleanser. This supplement's website simply declares: "Legislation prohibits us from talking about the herbs, however, there is a wealth of information available online on the uses of these over many years", so it doesn't actually tell potential customers anywhere what the combination is supposedly good for. Needless to say the tub doesn't mention that it should be avoided by those trying to conceive;

- curcumin with added MitoQ – a mitochondria-targeted anti-oxidant developed and patented in New Zealand in the 1990s. It is promoted for skincare and in a range of anti-oxidant supplements targeted at various body organs. With curcumin in this product, it is said to support "normal immune response pathways and key organ health, including the brain and the digestive system".

You can also find curcumin in a "natural blackcurrant flavour drink to help when you are feeling down in the dumps". Here 100mg of curcumin is combined with an assortment of vitamins, magnesium, zinc, quercitin (a plant polyphenol which demonstrates anti-oxidant activity *in vitro*) and tryptophan (an amino acid found in most protein-based foods).

Inevitably finding the right remedy to suit a particular ailment may involve sampling a range of turmeric extracts to find one that proves the most effective. That can be an expensive business given the price of many curcumin supplements: £20–£30 for a month's supply is not unusual. Such trial and error may even involve following the advice given by the manufacturer quoted earlier that suggested taking a couple of black peppercorns with the remedy to see if that improves the efficacy ... but somehow that doesn't really seem to improve confidence in the product. With so many different food supplements to choose from selecting an appropriate and effective turmeric remedy can clearly prove challenging.

Chapter 5

Curcumin vs turmeric

For anyone planning to try taking turmeric for health problems, the available choices can be bewildering:

- Should you choose a curcumin extract or simply ground
  turmeric?
- Should you opt for curcumin or focus on a curcuminoid mixture?
- Will turmeric's oils form an important therapeutic component?
- How do you balance claimed bioavailability with curcuminoid content?
- Which product would be best for arthritic problems? Which
  for depression? Digestive or skin problems?
- Should you add black pepper to whatever you decide to take?
      ... and much more. Small wonder so many online blogs and
  websites devoted to turmeric focus on the options available
  and recommend a preferred brand.

From what we now know of turmeric's constituents – all 235 of them – and the nature of curcumin, it is very difficult to be 100% certain in claiming that curcumin is the only constituent of any significance. Some studies, for example, have suggested that demethoxycurcumin is a more effective anti-inflammatory that curcumin. So, for example, opting for a curcuminoid rather than a pure curcumin extract may be preferable if the remedy is designed to treat an inflammatory problem, such as arthritis. Also, as discussed earlier, while much of the curcumin passes through the gut unchanged, some breaks down to produce new chemicals – phase-2 metabolites – which are eventually absorbed into the blood stream. These also show therapeutic properties, so, are they contributing to the perceived therapeutic effects of curcumin?

Turmeric's volatile oil component also has therapeutic effects and is regarded as a potential antibiotic[1], as well as having anti-inflammatory properties and has proved effective in studies involving arthritic rats[2]. So perhaps a remedy containing turmerones could be a good choice if the health problem involves any sort of infection or inflammation?

Which is best?

Patenting extracts from a particular herb is how plant extract producers and pharmaceutical companies make their money and cover the development costs of their products. So it is not surprising that most of the research into turmeric focusses on the action of individual constituents that can be isolated or synthesised, while the number of clinical trials using patented extracts far exceeds those involving basic turmeric rhizomes.

The poor oral absorption of curcumin is well-established, hence the emphasis by extract producers on improving bio-availability. Recent negative publicity about the effectiveness of curcumin may also have encouraged a tendency in marketing to focus on "turmeric" rather than "curcumin" – as with Cambridge Nutraceuticals renaming its curcumin-phospholipid product "Turmeric+". As Bill Zuercher, a chemical biologist at the University of North Carolina, commented in Nature's report of the extensive review of curcumin chemistry discussed earlier[3]: "It may very well be the case that curcumin or turmeric extracts do have beneficial effects, but getting to the bottom of that is complex and might be impossible"[4].

The various attempts to improve bioavailability by extract producers has clearly had an effect on the efficacy of their products, but since it is difficult to know for certain that curcumin – and only curcumin – is the key constituent it is difficult to understand just what the various claims about bioavailability really mean. Those early experiments with rats[5] suggested that 75% of ingested curcumin was excreted in the faeces. Equally, Cambridge Nutraceuticals argues that 99.8% of basic curcumin "disintegrates in the stomach" to form those phase-2 metabolites – which could be taken to imply that only 0.2% remains to be absorbed unchanged into the blood stream.

But, if the bulk of the curcumin taken in a capsule breaks down to form other chemicals, then why did those researchers back in the 1970s find so much unchanged curcumin in the rats' droppings? And if so little curcumin – 0.2% of any that is ingested – is actually available to be absorbed, then what does increasing bioavailability by × 7, × 30 or even × 185 actually mean? 185 × 0.2% = 37% – so does that mean that this particular extract allows a little more than a third of the curcumin provided to enter the blood stream unchanged? Small wonder the whole area is fraught with confusion.

If curcumin is the single vital ingredient then it would seem that very high doses of turmeric would have been needed in the past by traditional healers in order to deliver a therapeutic effect. As discussed earlier, a modern medical herbalist may prescribe around 8g of turmeric powder daily, containing perhaps 360mg of curcumin. If 75% of any of the curcumin in the ingested turmeric powder is excreted that could leave somewhere around 90mg of curcumin that may be absorbed (even as break-down products) into the system. In contrast many patented curcumin food supplements deliver a total of little more than 40mg of curcumin daily – although they do promise much greater bioavailability. It is perhaps also worth noting that aqueous extracts of turmeric containing neither essential oils nor curcumin still have an anti-inflammatory effect,[6] which does rather suggest that other chemicals in turmeric, not only curcumin, might be rather useful.

Turmeric side effects

As a traditional culinary herb, moderate use of turmeric is likely to produce few side effects and it is generally regarded as safe at the sort of dosage recommended by the food supplement producers. These dosages tend to be rather lower than those used in many clinical trials involving curcumin, although even those using high dosages generally report that the extract was still well tolerated. Problems can arise with prolonged use of higher than average doses or in certain medical conditions.

The German "Commission E" monograph[7] only warns that turmeric is contraindicated in any obstructions of the biliary tract (i.e. liver, gall bladder and bile ducts) and recommends seeking professional advice if gallstones are present. This is perhaps a little curious given that studies involving mice have demonstrated that turmeric actually reduced bile duct blockages.

As with several other herbs turmeric also demonstrates anti-platelet activity so should not be used when taking blood-thinning medication, such as heparin or warfarin, or if there are any bleeding disorders or after surgery. If taking turmeric as a long-term supplement it is best to stop at least two weeks before any elective surgery is planned. Many herbs have a high salicylate content – similar to aspirin – and these can also slow blood clotting so care needs to be taken if using turmeric with other salicylate-containing herbs.

Clinical trials involving higher doses of turmeric or curcumin (1g a day or more) do occasionally report that a small number of patients dropped out due to adverse gastro-intestinal effects including nausea, vomiting, stomach upsets, and diarrhoea. There are also anecdotal reports of allergic reactions to turmeric involving dermatitis and skin irritation, although these appear to be rare. As it is a member of the ginger family, it is also best avoided by anyone who is allergic to ginger.

Animal studies have suggested that turmeric can stimulate uterine muscle so therapeutic doses are probably best avoided in pregnancy, although in Fiji, turmeric is traditionally taken after childbirth to encourage milk flow in the new mother. The amount generally used in cooking in regarded as quite safe during pregnancy.

Studies suggest that curcumin can reduce blood sugar levels[8] so, although it has been used in a number of clinical trials involving diabetic patients with positive results, it needs to be used with caution by diabetics as it may impact their management of blood sugar levels. Turmeric has also been shown to cause hair loss in rats and is traditionally used in India as a paste to remove unwanted facial hair, so turmeric should probably also be used cautiously by anyone suffering from thinning hair or hair loss.

Turmeric has a high oxalate content, and one study has demonstrated that it significantly increases the levels of oxalates excreted in urine, so it should be avoided or used with caution by anyone at risk of kidney stones[9].

Some legalities

Under the rules of the EU's Directive on Traditional Herbal Medicinal Products the claims that producers of herbal remedies can make for their products are severely restricted. A company must demonstrate that the herb has been "in use within the EU for at least 30 years or 15 years within the EU and 30 years outside the EU", while herbal medicine products manufactured using "isolated active ingredients from plants" will not be regarded as herbal medicines and will not receive an authorisation under this scheme.

As noted earlier, herbal texts of 15 or 30 years ago offered very limited applications for turmeric. The Commission E monograph dating from 1985 and revised in 1990, lists only "dyspeptic conditions" as a use for turmeric. Even in 2000, the list of European uses for turmeric was limited to little more than "rheumatoid arthritis, osteoarthritis, dyspepsia, poor digestion and topically for skin lesions".

This means that under the 30 year rule, turmeric products cannot make any claims for efficacy beyond these basic lists without extensive clinical trials or well-supported evidence of approved clinical use elsewhere (i.e. 30 years of similar use in India to that claimed for 15 years in the EU). Similarly, since curcumin is beyond the scope of the THMP directive, it also needs extensive research results in order to be licensed as a "drug" and make specific claims for efficacy. Hence, all those products simply sold as "food supplements" with little indication on the tubs as to what they might be good for.

Personal preferences

In today's social media age, food supplement websites generally list dozens of satisfied reviews from customers reporting instant relief from their aches and pains by taking particular brands of curcumin extract. If that is the case then that is great for the patients and there is no reason why they should stop taking their preferred capsules.

However, not all consumer reviews on food supplement websites are equally eulogising and many come into the "no improvement yet" category. Curcumin extracts can be expensive – even more so if you have to keep trying different ones to see which work for you. In contrast, a spoonful of powder or freshly grated turmeric root infused in hot milk, is not. Given the many questions over the stability and degradation of curcumin, as well as the demonstrated therapeutic attributes of its other chemical constituents, there are good arguments for trying the whole herb instead.

There is, of course, the little matter of the placebo effect. With some ailments it is recognised that up to 40% of patients can be placebo responders while a recent report[10] which involved actually telling patients they were taking a placebo, found that subjects responded equally well to the actual medication used in the trial as to the known placebo. If placebos work for you – well done! You will avoid the side effects of all sorts of drugs by taking something totally innocuous that you believe works.

Chapter 6

All sorts of uses: fact or fiction?

Some of the claims made for turmeric and curcumin – as listed in the opening chapter – would appear to suggest that it really is a universal panacea: capable of "curing" anything from arthritis to Alzheimer's, cancer to Crohn's, diabetes to depression . . . and a great many more. If it performed half the miracles claimed for it, then surely it could bring an end to all of humankind's ills.

Sadly, fact is rather different from marketing fiction. Turmeric and/or curcumin can certainly live up to many of the claims made – but the results of limited controlled trials, which even the authors admit are inconclusive, are regularly exaggerated and the scientists' cautious provisos conveniently ignored. There have been a number of critical reviews and studies in the past couple of years trying to separate reality from hype and many of these have already been referred to: details can be found in "Notes and references" at the end of this book.

So just what can anyone expect from those many thousands

of tubs containing curcumin or turmeric capsules that fill the health food shop shelves?

Turmeric as anti-inflammatory

There have been numerous studies since the 1970s – animal and *in vitro* as well as clinical trials – that have demonstrated the anti-inflammatory properties of curcumin. In animal studies aqueous extracts of whole turmeric (i.e. not containing curcumin) have also shown "cortisone-like" anti-inflammatory activity[1]. In traditional medicine turmeric used for topical application (i.e. external use) was often mixed with slaked lime, which would have increased the water solubility of curcumin by forming a salt of the chemical. Researchers have tested sodium curcuminate in this way and found that it demonstrated much higher anti-inflammatory activity in rats than curcumin or hydrocortisone[2].

There have also been several clinical trials using different curcumin extracts which have demonstrated efficacy in treating both rheumatoid arthritis and osteoarthritis. A recent review by Kunnumakkara *et al.*[3] listed seven clinical trials using curcumin extracts for osteoarthritis held between 2010 and 2014 and all of them demonstrated various degrees of efficacy at doses between 180mg and 1.5g daily. Two trials involving a small number of rheumatoid arthritis patients in 1980 and 2012 also showed a reduction in symptoms. Taking either turmeric or curcumin extracts internally, or applying a traditional turmeric-based mixture externally to arthritic joints, would thus appear to be effective options for treating arthritic conditions.

Clinical trials have also covered a wide range of other inflammatory disorders – from gingivitis and periodontitis to pancreatitis and Crohn's disease. In most cases some improvement in symptoms is claimed, although a few recorded no significant effects. Some of these trials are referred to in the following sections where relevant.

Turmeric as anti-oxidant

Anti-oxidants – as the name implies – inhibit the oxidation of molecules. Within the body oxidation can produce free radicals: these are atoms, molecules or ions (charged particles), which contain an unpaired valence electron, that is, an extra electron that is looking for another atom, molecule or ion to interact with. The result is chain reactions which damage cells. Free radicals are generally regarded in the popular health press as highly damaging and requiring a raft of dietary supplements to combat them. However, animals, as well as humans, produce a number of anti-oxidants naturally; these include uric acid, glutathione, melatonin, and – for all animals except humans and guinea pigs – vitamin C: one vitamin that we all sometimes need to take as an additional supplement. Other anti-oxidants, such as vitamin E, are largely obtained from dietary sources.

Oxidation – like inflammation – is recognised as a significant causal factor in many chronic conditions and as a result, many food supplements are promoted as anti-oxidants and claim to improve general health, combat ageing, and prevent several degenerative and chronic disorders including heart disease, cancer, Alzheimer's or Parkinson's disease. However, trials using anti-oxidant supplements as preventatives have generally proved inconclusive.

Polyphenols are found in all plants and many anti-oxidant supplements are derived from these chemicals. Several show some anti-oxidant properties *in vitro* but, as they break down rapidly in the digestive system, may or may not perform the same function *in vivo*. Curcumin – a polyphenol – is no exception. Numerous *in vitro* studies have demonstrated its anti-oxidant activity, as have a few uncontrolled trials (where the action of the test material is not compared with placebo). Aqueous turmeric extracts (i.e. not containing curcumin) have also demonstrated anti-oxidant activity[4], so – again – simply adding turmeric to food or taking the powder could be as effective as curcumin capsules.

Turmeric as anti-microbial

Various turmeric extracts, its essential oils, and the curcuminoids have all demonstrated anti-microbial activity *in vitro* – again, this doesn't mean the same thing happens *in vivo* as plant constituents break down in the stomach or may be excreted as waste matter. However, in traditional medicine, turmeric has long been used for conditions associated with infection including fevers, cholera, and syphilis. Its traditional use against scabies also suggests anti-parasitic properties, while putting a pinch of turmeric powder on a cut or graze to prevent infection and encourage healing is a long-standing household remedy in India. See also Postscript p.133.

Studies *in vitro* with curcumin have found that low levels are effective against *Salmonella* spp. in the presence of visible light, which suggests that the breakdown products – those phase-2 metabolites again – have anti-microbial properties[5]. Turmeric extracts have also proved effective against MRSA (Methicillin-resistant *Staphylococcus aureus*) *in vitro* and turmeric oil shows anti-fungal action in tests involving guinea pigs. In Kunnumakkara *et al.*'s review[3], one clinical trial using curcumin for HIV concluded only that it was "well tolerated", while a larger one involving 578 patients suffering from tuberculosis described the key clinical outcome as "prevented hepatotoxicity" – i.e. helped to prevent drug-induced liver damage.

A great many herbs, just like turmeric and its various chemical constituents, tested *in vitro* show anti-microbial action and perhaps many of them could prove valuable in future as antibiotic resistance increases. However, there is already a wide choice of effective anti-microbial herbs in use and many are readily available commercially in licensed products. Turmeric is certainly effective – but it may not be everyone's remedy of choice for cuts and grazes given its tendency to cause a yellow stain when used in creams or ointments.

With both anti-microbial and anti-oxidant activity it is perhaps not surprising that turmeric has also traditionally been used as a preservative, with several studies in recent years demonstrating that it helps prolong the shelf life of many foods. Some researchers have argued that the herb's use as a food preservative and culinary spice in Asian countries could help explain why there is a much lower incidence of childhood leukaemia in India, China and Japan compared with the USA and UK[6].

Turmeric for the digestion

Turmeric and other related *Curcuma* spp. have all traditionally been used for various digestive upsets including indigestion, diarrhoea, and as a bile stimulant. Early research studies have linked this activity to the essential oil, rather than curcumin, although sodium curcuminate (a salt of curcumin) also acts as a bile stimulant[7]. Many later studies have involved rats, mice, rabbits or *in vitro* experiments and have demonstrated that curcumin can help combat the effects of the *Helicobactor pylori* bacterium, now known as a prime cause of stomach ulcers. It also has an anti-spasmodic effect on the muscles of the gut so could ease cramping pains.

Clinical trials using curcumin for gastritis, peptic ulcers, and *H. pylori* infections have had mixed results – ranging from "no significant effect" to "alleviated abdominal pain and discomfort"[3] while the use of curcuminoid enemas for treating ulcerative colitis and Chrohn's disease appears to be have been more effective[3]. However, some of the trials have involved very few patients – occasionally as few as five or even, in one study, a solitary subject – and even the authors of a clinical trial involving 45 patients concluded that while curcumin performed better than placebo in terms of healing and outcome, the differences were not statistically significant[8].

There is little modern research into turmeric's traditional use as a carminative to ease indigestion, but many culinary herbs also have this property – which is perhaps one of the reasons why they have proved popular in cooking over the centuries. Similarly, one can speculate that the traditional use of turmeric in Eastern medicine for diarrhoea may have more to do with its anti-microbial activity in hot countries where epidemic disorders, such as cholera, have been commonplace, rather than being due to any physiological action on gut tissue.

Turmeric capsules sold as food supplements do sometimes advertise themselves as "digestive aids" and since this is a very long-standing and often quoted traditional use it is worth trying, although the same properties may not apply to curcumin taken on its own.

Turmeric for the liver

Curcumin hit the media headlines a few years ago when the *Daily Mirror* ran a story headed "Curry favour for your liver" based on an animal study that demonstrated that it has hepatoprotective properties (i.e. it helps to prevent damage to the liver). Studies[9] in 2010 using mice with chronic liver inflammation, demonstrated that a diet including curcumin significantly reduced bile duct blockage and curbed liver cell damage and scarring – possibly due to curcumin interfering with chemical processes that caused inflammation. A later clinical trial[10] involved giving curcumin to patients who had just had their gall bladders removed. It concluded that this "improved post-operative pain" – although one may have hoped that the researchers might have chosen to test the effect of giving curcumin to patients rather sooner, so that surgery might have been avoided.

As with its use in digestive disorders, turmeric is a traditional remedy for liver problems and has long been used for jaundice: this is a fairly commonplace association for herbs and spices that are yellow in colour, based on the old "doctrine of signatures" with the plant's appearance giving a clue to its therapeutic properties. However, both the 2010 mouse study and later research suggest that turmeric and/or curcumin can be useful for combatting various progressive inflammatory liver disorders, notably primary sclerosing cholangitis (where the bile ducts inside and outside the liver progressively decrease in size due to inflammation and scarring) and primary biliary cirrhosis (an autoimmune condition which damages the bile ducts) – both are conditions which can ultimately cause liver cirrhosis.

Other studies have confirmed that curcumin can help prevent damage to the liver caused by "ethanol, thioacetamide, iron overdose, cholestasis and acute, subchronic and chronic carbon tetrachloride intoxication"[11]; it may also reduce the risk of hepatitis (B and C), combat non-alcoholic fatty liver disorders, and may be helpful for some types of liver cancer[12] – although, as usual, many of these studies are *in vitro* with very few large scale clinical trials.

One recent study[13] found that a hot water extract of

turmeric helped to counter alcohol-induced liver damage in rats while, in the same study, another of turmeric's constituents, bisacurone, also proved effective. Since curcumin is not soluble in water it clearly did not contribute to this outcome. So far none of the curcumin extract makers appears to be actively promoting their products as suitable for combatting liver damage, but perhaps regularly using a little turmeric in cooking might just help maintain liver health.

The German "Commission E" monographs – which in the past tended to form the basis of EU recommendations on what you can and cannot say about a herb's properties – advise that turmeric root is contraindicated in: "Obstruction of bile passages (i.e. liver, gall bladder and bile ducts). In case of gallstones, use only after consulting with a physician"[14]. The WHO monograph on turmeric root gives a similar warning[15]. Both monographs date from the 1990s, and seem to contradict the findings that curcumin "significantly reduced bile duct blockage" in those mice experiments in 2010.

Turmeric and diabetes

The marketing material associated with some brands of curcumin and turmeric food supplements often claims that the product will help combat type 2 diabetes. Clinical trials suggest that there may be some truth in these claims with various studies reporting reduced blood glucose levels, raised insulin production and reduction in oxidative stress which can contribute to the condition. Almost all were small scale – one early report involved a single patient taking 5g of a curcumin extract a day for three months, for example[16].

A review in 2013 of studies – animal and human – that had used turmeric or curcumin to control diabetes[17] concluded: "Curcumin could favorably affect most of the leading aspects of

diabetes, including insulin resistance, hyperglycemia, hyperlipi-
demia, and islet apoptosis and necrosis. In addition, curcumin
could prevent the deleterious complications of diabetes …
Studies are badly needed to be done in humans to confirm
the potential of curcumin in limitation of diabetes and other
associated disorders".

According to Kunnumakkara *et al.*'s 2017 review of clinical
trials[3], only three involving curcumin extracts and diabetes
have been completed since 2013, with two more still ongoing,
so it could be many years before turmeric extracts become
widely accepted as a suitable treatment. Dosages used in
those trials where the findings have been published, vary
from 300mg to 5g per day. Most used a curcumin formulation,
but one with positive results used 500mg of turmeric three
times a day[18].

Using turmeric in cooking, or taking a turmeric supplement
may be helpful for those at risk of type 2 diabetes or where the
condition is being controlled by diet alone. For those already
on medication, careful monitoring of blood sugar levels may be
needed to ensure that they are not affected by doses of turmeric
adding to the drug-related therapeutics.

Turmeric and cholesterol

Views on cholesterol have varied significantly over the years:
from being something to avoid at all costs to the realisation
that perhaps it's not that bad after all. Cholesterol is essential
for various bodily functions and if we don't eat enough of it
then our internal chemical factory simply produces more.
Cholesterol forms a part of every cell membrane in our bodies,
is a vital ingredient for making steroid hormones and vitamin
D, and is also used to synthesise bile acids, which are important
for the digestion of fats.

Cholesterol travels through the blood stream in the form of lipoproteins either low-density lipoproteins (LDL) or high density lipoproteins (HDL). LDL is sometimes called "bad cholesterol" as too much of it can cause furring up of the arteries leading to atherosclerosis, while HDL is deemed "good cholesterol" because it carries cholesterol back to the liver where any surplus can be excreted.

Various studies with both turmeric and curcumin have demonstrated that it will reduce cholesterol levels in laboratory animals with one[19], involving rats, suggesting that while LDL levels in the blood were reduced by 42.5%, HDL-levels were increased by 50%. Another – using real people: 63 patients with acute coronary syndrome – found that low dose curcumin "showed a trend of reduction in total cholesterol level and LDL cholesterol level"[20], while a controlled trial with a total of 67 type 2 diabetes patients, found that a "NCB-02 – standardised preparation of curcuminoids"[21] had some beneficial effect in reducing oxidative stress – a condition associated with oxidising LDL and so causing that furring of the arteries. The authors of this one concluded that: "Further studies are needed to evaluate the potential long-term effects of NCB-02 and its combination with other herbal anti-oxidants"[22].

In contrast a study, based on 36 elderly subjects taking curcumin or placebo for six months, concluded that: "Curcumin consumption does not appear to have a significant effect on the serum lipid profile, unless the absorbed concentration of curcumin is considered, in which case curcumin may modestly increase cholesterol"[23].

So, as often happens with curcumin research, the findings appear indecisive and conflicting. Adding a little turmeric in cooking may be no bad thing, but if you are concerned about cholesterol levels and the associated risks of type 2 diabetes, avoiding dietary fats is not necessarily the answer[24].

Turmeric for neurological diseases

Curcumin extracts and turmeric have also been recommended for depression, anxiety and to combat Alzheimer's disease. Among the extract producers, both Verdure Sciences (Longvida®) and Arjuna (BCM-95®) have promoted their products for neurological problems. BCM-95® has been used in a series of trials, led by Adrian Loperesti, in Australia since 2012, which have apparently successfully reduced patients' symptoms[25]. Arjuna quotes Loperesti as saying: "Curcumin's positive anti-depressant and anti-anxiety effects are likely due to its ability to normalise specific physiological pathways. It appears to elevate neurotransmitters such as serotonin, while lowering stress hormones, such as cortisol, and is a potent anti-oxidant and anti-inflammatory. Curcumin also provides protection to the brain"[26].

Critics are not convinced: reviewing the Loperesti *et al.* trials, as well as several others, Dr Chittaranjan Andrade has pointed out that many of these trials have been small, poorly controlled, and used low doses of curcumin, while patients were often also taking prescription anti-depressants. He concluded that: "... controlled clinical trials provide no convincing evidence that patients with major depressive illness fare better with different extracts of curcumin (dosed at 500–1,000 mg/day) than with placebo (or no treatment) after 5–8 weeks of monotherapy or anti-depressant-augmentation therapy. At present, therefore, there is insufficient evidence to encourage depressed patients to consider curcumin as a possible alternative to standard anti-depressant therapy"[27].

In theory turmeric possesses the properties deemed likely to help prevent Alzheimer's sufferers: it is anti-oxidant, anti-inflammatory, may (or may not) help reduce cholesterol levels, while some studies suggest it can improve cognitive function in the elderly and research with rats has demonstrated that it will also chelate (trap and help to remove) heavy metals from the system – pollutants associated by some with Alzheimer's. *In vitro* studies also suggest that curcumin may help prevent the development of amyloid plaques also associated with Alzheimer's[28]. In addition aromatic turmerone – included in BCM-95® – has been shown to encourage the proliferation of neural stem cells, so potentially could be of use in repairing brain damage[29].

Two clinical trials involving Alzheimer's patients were reviewed by Kunnumakkara *et al.*[3]. One, dating from 2005 has yet to publish the patients' response, while the other which involved 34 patients given 1g or 4g daily for six months concluded: "Curcumin did not seem to cause side effects in Alzheimer's Disease patients (rather, there was a tendency toward fewer adverse events on 4g)" adding that "longer and larger trials to test the efficacy of curcumin" are needed. A more recent trial[30] involving 96 patients taking BCM-95®, concluded that: "... the results of the present study indicate that ... curcumin had limited influence on cognitive function, mood or general quality of life over 12 months" – again, the researchers also added that more long-term studies are needed.

Researchers are clearly hoping for better results: those involved in a 2012 trial[31] blamed bioavailability for failure: "Curcumin was generally well-tolerated ... we were unable to demonstrate clinical or biochemical evidence of efficacy of Curcumin C3 Complex(®) in Alzheimer's disease in this 24-week placebo-controlled trial although preliminary data suggest limited bioavailability of this compound".

Researchers have also investigated the association between curry consumption and cognitive level in 1,010 Asians between 60 and 93 years of age. The study found that those who occasionally ate curry (less than once a month) and often (more than once a month) performed better on a standard test of cognitive function than those who ate curry never or rarely[32]. However, not all curries contain turmeric and the amounts used in those that do often vary significantly between ethnic groups and geography. This group of researchers admitted that they didn't actually consider other dietary factors (fat, vegetable intake, additional herbs etc). Since curries are more likely to contain larger amounts of coriander, cumin and pepper than turmeric, perhaps these herbs might be worth investigating for their affect on cognitive function?

So turmeric (or curcumin) may or may not influence the development and progression of Alzheimer's – and the Alzheimer's Society currently regards the suggestion with caution: "Turmeric is not easily absorbed and there is no real evidence that supports turmeric being used as a treatment for Alzheimer's disease ... the evidence suggesting that turmeric may be beneficial when in the brain will make it a target for future research"[33]. See also p.133.

Turmeric and eye problems

In traditional Indian medicine turmeric is used to treat various eye disorders including hazy vision, eye inflammations and night blindness with turmeric paste applied directly to styes.

There have been very few clinical trials using curcumin extracts for eye problems although two small-scale projects involving the treatment of anterior uveitis (an inflammation of the uvea, the pigmented area of the eye that lies between the retina and the outer layer comprising sclera and cornea) did show positive benefits. One study in 1999[34] concluded that curcumin was equivalent to "giving corticosteroids" while in 2010 a second[35] found that it reduced symptoms and eye discomfort. Both involved small numbers of patients and the 2010 trial was uncontrolled, so would be deemed inconclusive, but if you suffer from anterior uveitis, taking regular doses of turmeric or a curcumin extract might just help.

There are suggestions[35] from *in vitro* studies in the USA that the plant may possibly also help prevent blindness caused by retinitis pigmentosa – a degenerative genetic condition affecting the rod photoreceptor cells in the retina – although research is still in the very early stages.

Turmeric and cancer

Much has also been written about turmeric's role in preventing and treating various cancers, although much is also anecdotal. In 2009 a group of Spanish doctors wrote to the *International Journal of Cancer*[37] voicing their concerns about claims made for curcumin in cancer treatments. Under the heading "*The dark side of curcumin*" the doctors argued that much of the research purporting to demonstrate that curcumin was active against cancer cells was *in vitro* and involved exposing the cells to curcumin for very long periods.

They argued that since curcumin degrades in the digestive tract it was never likely to be in contact with tumours within the body for the requisite amount of time to have any effect. They cited[38] a 2009 study which had carefully monitored plasma levels of curcumin in 12 healthy volunteers at regular intervals from 15 minutes to 72 hours after an oral dose of 10g or 12g of turmeric: only one of the subjects had detectable free curcumin in their system at any point in the trial. As the Spanish doctors said: "The fact that curcumin also undergoes extensive metabolism in intestine and liver means that high concentrations of curcumin cannot be achieved and maintained in plasma and tissues after oral ingestion. This is a major obstacle for the clinical development of this agent and suggests that the therapeutic potential of oral curcumin is limited".

While much repeated anecdotal evidence of cancer sufferers being helped by both turmeric and curcumin extracts
is regularly found on the Internet, clinical evidence of efficacy remains minimal. The numerous clinical trials typically
involve very few patients and the most common "clinical
outcome" recorded in a recent review of clinical trials[3] was
"safe and well-tolerated". Results also tend to be inconsistent.
For example, the reviewers included two trials using curcumin
to treat prostate cancer. One in 2010 involving 85 patients
suggested a significant reduction in levels of prostate specific
antigen (PSA) – an indicator of the likelihood of the presence
of cancerous cells – while a second trial in 2016 involving 40
patients found that curcumin had "no significant effect".

There are some suggestions that curcumin may enhance
the effectiveness of chemotherapy and other bowel cancer
treatments[39] and a study involving mice suggested that it may
prevent the spread of breast cancer cells to other parts of the
body[40]. However, as Cancer Research UK concludes: "... currently there is no conclusive research evidence to show that
turmeric or curcumin can prevent or treat cancer"[41].

Turmeric and curcumin, however, continue to be used in
cancer treatments among alternative healthcare providers.
I was told of one clinic in Germany which gives curcumin
extracts by injection combined with focussing bright light
on the vein being injected. Since curcumin degrades rapidly
in daylight, this could increase the presence of degradation
products which, as discussed earlier, appear to have significant
therapeutic properties.

Turmeric and viruses

Inevitably – like many other herbs – turmeric and curcumin
have been investigated in the past as potential anti-virals for

use in treating HIV (human immunodeficiency virus). *In vitro* curcumin demonstrates significant anti-viral activity against a range of pathogens including HIV, dengue virus, HPV (human papilloma virus which is often the cause of cervical cancer) and hepatitis C virus, while an aqueous extract (i.e. without curcumin) demonstrated anti-viral activity against hepatitis B virus[42].

More recently another *in vitro* study found that curcumin was active against Zika and chikungunya viruses, two mosquito-borne outbreak viruses[43]. Much of the research effort is concerned with understanding the anti-viral mechanism which is, as yet, not fully understood, although one group of researchers did suggest that "Curcumin in the human diet . . . could provide a simple means to prevent infection by enveloped viruses"[44]. Curcumin is, however, poorly absorbed and some of the researchers[45] have focussed attention on the breakdown products of curcumin or other chemicals derived from curcumin in an effort to identify potential future anti-viral drugs.

It is, however, a very long way from *in vitro* discovery to developing an anti-viral treatment based on turmeric extracts and the only relevant clinical trial, so far, was reported back in 1996 involving 40 HIV patients with the conclusion that curcumin at 2.5g per day was "well tolerated" and after eight weeks the patients "felt better" although there was no reduction in viral load.[46]

Turmeric for skin disorders

Turmeric has long been associated with beautiful skin and in some parts of India it was believed that if women ate plenty of turmeric during pregnancy then their child would be guaranteed a lovely complexion. Using it to stain the skin a light golden colour is also highly regarded in some cultures – although probably not among the pallid faces of ethnic northern Europeans who would probably be suspected of suffering from jaundice.

Because curcumin and/or turmeric tend to be used topically for skin conditions the problems associated with chemical degradation and bioavailability are no longer as significant and many clinical trials or case reports record high success levels. In trials curcumin cream has proved effective for vitiligo[47] while a US study found that 70% of 647 psoriasis patients improved when curcumin gel (1%) was combined with steroids. A more concentrated curcumin gel has helped reduce scarring after surgery, rosacea and UV-induced skin inflammations.[48]

Several clinical trials have also reported a degree of success with patients taking curcumin internally (up to 4.5g daily) for psoriasis, although the trials have been small, comparatively short and uncontrolled so further research is needed.[3] A review of 234 research studies using turmeric or curcumin for skin disorders found that either topical, oral or a combination of both, could be helpful for acne, alopecia, atopic dermatitis, facial photoageing, oral lichen planus, pruritus, psoriasis, radiodermatitis, and vitiligo.[49]

One study, involving mice and human cancer cells *in vitro*, found that using a topical curcumin cream for skin squamous cell carcinoma – one of the most common skin cancers – was just as effective as taking oral curcumin. The researchers also suggested that topical curcumin may have a role as a preventative treatment[50]. Ayurvedic practitioners also suggest turmeric capsules as a preventative for melanoma and using a paste made from 1 part turmeric to 2 parts ghee as a sun block for moles.[51]

• Methods of making your own turmeric cream or ointment can be found in Appendix 3.

Turmeric for cardiovascular problems

Both turmeric and curcumin are often suggested by supplement producers as preventatives for heart disease. This tends to be because of the herb's anti-cholesterol, anti-inflammatory and anti-oxidant activities since high lipid levels, oxidation and inflammation are among causal factors for heart problems. Studies usually focus on the effect curcumin has on blood vessels – one Japanese study measured the effect of eating curry on endothelial function[52] (the way the inner lining of blood vessels behaves with dysfunction ultimately leading to atherosclerosis and coronary heart disease), while another trial has tested whether curcuminoids reduced the risk of heart attacks following bypass surgery[53]. Both studies claimed positive results, although the sample sizes were small (14 and 121 respectively).

Interestingly, the Japanese group which looked at the effect of eating curry give their curry spice mix per serving as: "cloves 0.9g, coriander 1.8g, cumin 0.9g, garlic 3.6g, ginger 2.7g, onion (sautéed) 9g, red pepper 0.09g and turmeric 4.5g". Typically a teaspoon of powdered spice weighs about 4–5g so the "recipe" made a curry with barely a quarter of a teaspoon (1g) for cloves and cumin, under a half for coriander and a whole teaspoon of turmeric powder per serving – which is significantly disproportional to the spices many cooks would use.

Turmeric for good health

Given the various rules about the claims food supplement manufacturers can and cannot make for their products in the UK and Europe, tubs of curcumin and turmeric capsules only make vague suggestions as to why the spice may be beneficial. Turmeric products sometimes mention that it is good for the digestion, while curcumin capsules may hint at anti-oxidant and anti-inflammatory properties.

As already discussed, both oxidation and inflammation can contribute to a range of health problems and the two conditions are also linked[54] with free radicals – produced by oxidation – involved with oxidative stress, which can then lead to inflammation. Inflammation can also increase production of free radicals, as the white blood cells that try to combat inflammation also leave free radicals in their wake. Dietary sources and normal metabolism, providing such anti-oxidants as vitamin E and glutathione, help to keep both conditions under control but specific herbs and spices can also provide extra support.

Turmeric is certainly good at combatting both conditions, but so too are a great many other herbs, including several that are also used in cooking. The list of anti-inflammatories, for example, includes: bilberry, black cohosh, black pepper, boswellia, chamomile, Chinese angelica, echinacea, evening primrose oil, eyebright, fenugreek, garlic, ginger, globe artichoke, gotu kola, hawthorn, liquorice, marigold, meadowsweet, peppermint, saffron, St John's wort, stinging nettle, thyme, and willow bark – to name just a few.

Anti-oxidant herbs include: basil, black pepper, cinnamon, cloves, coriander, cumin, fennel, garlic, ginger, oregano, parsley, rosemary, sage, thyme, and walnuts – again this list is also far from complete.

Turmeric is certainly up there with the best of them in both categories, but if you are looking for herbs to improve health and act as a preventative, then the immune-stimulating ones should also be added: such as, ashwagandha, astragalus, Chinese angelica, echinacea, ginseng, liquorice, meadowsweet, milk thistle, Siberian ginseng – plus numerous mushrooms and fungi, such as shiitake, maitake and reishi.

As always a balanced diet, including plenty of fresh fruits and vegetables, good quality protein sources and fats, should be delivering a healthy sprinkling of anti-inflammatories and anti-oxidants – as well as all those vital vitamins, minerals, amino acids and essential fatty acids. For healthy individuals, additional supplements should not really be needed, although they can of course be helpful for the debilitated or those suffering from chronic illnesses or metabolic disorders.

Using herbs in cooking and making herbal teas and other therapeutic drinks instead of popping pills, can deliver many benefits – as can eating curry. It is also worth remembering that not all curries contain turmeric and that many Indian cooks regard the turmeric component as mainly there to add colour, with the real flavour coming from the other spices used – and some of those also have significant therapeutic properties.

Chapter 7

Spice up your menu

With suggestions that eating curry may enhance cognitive function[1] in the elderly and that turmeric can protect the liver and improve joint health, it is not surprising that numerous recipes for turmeric drinks and various "healthy eating" dishes using turmeric can be found online and regularly appear in the media. Ground turmeric is readily available in supermarkets and whole rhizomes – fresh or dried – can be found in some supermarkets or from specialist suppliers. In many geographies where it is grown turmeric rhizome is dried immediately after harvest, however, in Thailand turmeric is generally used fresh so companies selling Thai cooking ingredients usually have fresh rhizomes available.

While it is not especially expensive – you can buy 1kg of turmeric powder for about £7 and whole rhizomes for about £1.50–£2 per 100g – quality can vary. As noted earlier, there have been numerous reports of medicinal grade curcumin being adulterated with the synthetic variety, while culinary grade turmeric is often mixed with fillers dyed yellow. Buying from a reputable source is obviously essential – if in doubt use the dried or fresh rhizomes.

Turmeric drinks

As discussed earlier, some of turmeric's key constituents – the curcuminoids and turmerones – are fat soluble so making turmeric drinks with some sort of milk rather than water alone could improve their extraction. This is obviously an important consideration for those that believe curcumin is the key to turmeric's therapeutic properties. Turmeric extracts made with hot water can also help repair liver damage[2] so, even a basic decoction will include some therapeutic constituents. Some suggest using a vegetable or meat stock to make turmeric tea, which would provide additional nutrients for anyone suffering from debility.

"Golden milk" or *haldi ka doodh* can be made very simply by simmering half a teaspoon of good quality turmeric powder with a cup of 50:50 full fat milk and water for around 15–20 minutes. This is very similar to the way many in India make a normal tea drink with the leaves heated in milk and water rather than infused in a teapot before adding milk to the cup, as in Britain. Turmeric powder will not all dissolve so the mixture needs to be stirred well and drunk quickly to avoid leaving too much turmeric in the dregs at the bottom of the cup. Adding some freshly ground pepper may improve the bioavailability of any curcumin extracted in the process.

Recipes for numerous variants are readily available. Some substitute a thick slice of fresh turmeric rhizome for the powder and recommend adding a piece of cinnamon stick (or cinnamon powder) and slice of ginger root (or ginger powder) to the milk mixture before heating, others may use whole black peppercorns instead of ground. These mixtures obviously need to be strained before drinking. Ginger and cinnamon share some of turmeric's therapeutic properties as well as adding considerably to the flavour of the drink.

Others recipe writers suggest adding coconut oil, honey, maple syrup, a pinch of cayenne powder, cardamom, cloves, vanilla extract, or allspice, while one over-the-counter turmeric tea blend adds *lo han guo (Siraitia grosvenorii)* – a type of gourd growing in southern China, which is 300 times sweeter than sugar and is used in folk remedies for coughs and feverish conditions. These various strongly flavoured additions suggest that "golden milk" is not to everyone's taste.

As golden milk is often recommended by healthy eating enthusiasts, they sometimes stipulate raw (unpasteurised) dairy milk or, alternatively, coconut, soya or almond milk. Which you choose is largely a matter of taste preference or dictated by food intolerance or allergy – the choice is very unlikely to have a significant effect on the therapeutics of the drink.

One recipe, described in *The Times of India* as "authentic Ayurvedic"[3] suggests using turmeric rhizome as "the chances of contamination in the powder are high" and recommends the "variety used in cooking; *varali manjal* in Thamizh".

1   Take an inch-long stick of turmeric and crush it coarsely using a pestle and mortar.
2   Crush a few peppercorns: "The white variety is better".
3   Mix a cup of water with a cup of milk, add the crushed turmeric and pepper and bring to the boil.
4   Simmer for 20 minutes. By this time, the quantity will reduce to one cup.
5   Strain, add a spoonful of honey or palm sugar, and drink warm.

The recipe adds that if the turmeric drink is being taken for a sore throat "add half a teaspoon of ghee".

An alternative to simmering all the ingredients together is to make turmeric paste. The simplest way is to mix:

2 tablespoons of powdered turmeric
½ teaspoon of ground pepper
5fl oz / 140ml of water
3fl oz / 85ml olive oil or ghee

Put the turmeric and water into a small pan and mix well. Cook gently over a low heat stirring all the time to produce a paste. Add the pepper and olive oil or ghee and stir well in. Store in a small jar in the refrigerator where it will last for about a week.

This can then be used to make the golden milk by combining:

½ teaspoon turmeric paste
5fl oz / 140ml milk (dairy, coconut, soya, almond – whatever your preference)
1 teaspoon of oil (e.g. coconut, olive, or almond) or ghee

In a saucepan heat gently for about 10 minutes or until the paste is well dispersed in the milk. Do not allow the mixture to boil. You can also heat with half a teaspoon of ground cinnamon and/or ground ginger to taste, as well as adding a teaspoon of honey before drinking.

Many recipes for golden milk and similar turmeric-based drinks can be rather confusing – some call for "turmeric juice" or "turmeric sprigs". "Turmeric sprigs" remains a mystery to me – perhaps the original recipe called for "turmeric root, mint sprigs" and some vital words were lost in the print and production process? "Sprigs" suggest parts of the fresh plant, such as a leaf of flower stem. As turmeric grows in tropical regions it may be easy to obtain these at certain times of year and they are used in Thai cooking. Elsewhere it is possible to grow turmeric indoors in a large pot but that is hardly going to provide a regular supply of "sprigs" for tea making.

"Turmeric juice" is a more variable entity. It has been used in traditional medicine as drops for eye complaints and can be made at home by processing turmeric rhizomes, and then the discharged pulp, through a juicer three or four times as the yield is not great. It will last for about three days if kept in the refrigerator. Rather than attempting to drink the pure juice – which in large quantities may cause gastric upsets and other side effects – it is generally well diluted with water or apple juice and flavoured with lemon, ginger and/or honey. "Turmeric juice" in some contexts can also be a mixture of a small amount of turmeric, with black pepper and sometimes ginger root, combined in a juicer with a combination of fruit and vegetables, such as apples, pears, oranges, celery, lemons or carrots.

Commercial "turmeric juice" drinks may be largely apple or pineapple juice with around 10–15% turmeric juice obtained from cold pressing the fresh root. One claims to contain "filtered water 88%, almonds 8%, coconut nectar 3%, ginger 1%, turmeric, black pepper". Since the quantified ingredients add up to 100% one is left wondering just how much turmeric and black pepper there may be in the mix, with the turmeric possibly added purely as a colouring agent – in which case why black pepper as well?

Another, rather more expensive, turmeric juice drink lists its ingredients as "organic turmeric purée – 99.5% (whole root), triple filtered water, organic stevia, citric acid, black pepper and potassium sorbate" – once again pepper is there to presumably enhance bioavailability.

Turmeric in curry powder

While turmeric is generally associated with curry in the West, that tends to be because commercial curry powders contain a high proportion of the spice, whereas not all curries from Southeast Asia contain turmeric and those that do have very variable amounts. Thai curry paste, for example, usually contains shrimp paste, red or green peppers (depending on the paste), onions or shallots, garlic, lemongrass, galangal and coriander; yellow Thai curry paste contain turmeric but green or red ones may not.

Malaysian curries generally have a high proportion of turmeric along with shrimp paste, tamarind, shallots, ginger, coconut milk, chilli peppers and garlic, while rogan josh from Kashmir is likely to be coloured red from chilli peppers and cockscomb flowers (*Celosia cristata*) or alkanet (*Alkanna tinctoria*), rather than yellow from turmeric.

Curry powder was an invention of the British Raj – perhaps one of the earliest forms of convenience food – enabling those returning from work in India to easily recreate the spicy dishes to which they had become accustomed. Traditionally the spices used for the curry would have been freshly ground when required for maximum flavour and freshness, thus any turmeric included would have been used before the curcumin content began to degrade in sunlight. Once ground any remaining curry spice mixture should be stored in a cool dry place away from direct sunlight and in a small air-tight container.

There are probably as many recipes for curry powder as there are different types of curry and the proportion of turmeric used can vary from around 5% to 20% or more. A very basic mixture might be:

8 parts ground coriander
4 parts ground cumin
1 part ground turmeric
1 part cayenne powder

or perhaps a mixture to be ground together, such as:

2 parts cumin seeds
1 part coriander seeds,
1 part white peppercorns,
1 part cayenne powder
1 part turmeric root
½ part fenugreek seeds.

While another recipe includes:

9 parts ground coriander
4 parts ground turmeric
3 parts ground cumin
1 part ground black pepper
1 part cayenne powder
1 part ground cardamon
1 part ground cinnamon
½ part ground cloves
½ part ground ginger
½ part fenugreek seeds.

The permutations really are endless and since manufacturers of curry powder give very little information on the side of their packs about the proportions of spices used in the mixture anyone expecting to eat a reasonable amount of turmeric in a curry using commercial curry powder may be disappointed. Possibly up to two or three tablespoons of curry powder – depending on the variety used and personal preferences – might be added to a curry to serve four people so with some mixtures the amount of turmeric per person may be very small. Eating curry with a high-turmeric content curry powder every day might boost intake – but it is just as easy to add spices individually to the dish. One also needs to be careful to balance the flavour of turmeric, which can give a rather bitter taste to a dish if used in excess.

While many curries often include cayenne or chilli pepper, this only arrived in India from South America with the Portuguese in Goa in the 1500s, before that pepper would probably have been the hottest spice used – ideal to enhance the bioavailability of any curcumin in the curry mix.

Turmeric in cooking

Turmeric can, of course, be added to plenty of other sorts of dishes, not only curries. It has long been used as a cheap alternative to saffron for colouring rice and it is still sometimes called *safran des Indes* in France. The result lacks saffron's delicate flavour but delivers a strong yellow colour and the taste of the turmeric does not dominate if you don't add too much. Marco Polo is often credited with being the first European to record turmeric's use in this way: "There is a fruit here that resembles saffron; though it is nothing of the sort, it is quite as good as saffron for practical purposes . . ."[4]. "Fruit" is sometimes translated as "vegetable" but neither seems very much like a description of turmeric rhizome and scholars suggest that Polo was actually describing either bastard saffron, (*Carthamus tinctorius*) or a type of gardenia fruit used in China for colouring. According to Hanbury, gardenia's yellow colour "is due to a body named crocine which appears to be identical with the polychroite of saffron"[5].

To make turmeric rice, simply stir ½–1 teaspoon of ground turmeric into your rice pan when you start to cook. I add 1 teaspoon when cooking sufficient rice for about four portions and this gives a rich saffron-like colour, although some recipes specify half a teaspoon to that amount of rice.

You can also add turmeric to soups, stir fries, vegetable dishes and spicy meat or fish main meals. Here are a few suggestions.

Butternut, apple and turmeric soup

1 onion, peeled and finely sliced
1 medium-sized butternut squash, peeled, deseeded and cubed
1–2 eating apples, peeled cored and chopped
1 litre of vegetable bouillon (made up from powder or stock cube, or home-made vegetable stock if you prefer)
½ teaspoon ground coriander
½–1 teaspoon ground turmeric (according to taste)
1 tablespoon olive oil
salt and freshly ground black pepper
Cream (or crème fraîche) and chopped parsley to garnish (optional)

In a large saucepan, sauté the onion in the olive oil for 2–3 minutes until it colours, add the apple, coriander and turmeric and cook for a further 2–3 minutes. Add the butternut squash and bouillon or stock and bring to the boil, then lower the heat, cover and simmer for about 20 minutes or until the squash is soft and well cooked. Remove from the heat and use a stick blender to process the mixture into a smooth soup. Check the seasoning and add a little black pepper. Serve with a spoonful of cream (or crème fraîche) and parsley as a garnish if desired.

Spicy lentil soup

8oz/225g red lentils
1 medium onion, finely sliced
1 garlic clove, peeled and crushed
1 tablespoon tomato purée
½ teaspoon ground coriander seeds
½ teaspoon ground cumin
½ teaspoon crushed mustard seeds
½ teaspoon ground turmeric
1 litre of vegetable bouillon (made up from powder or stock
    cube, or home-made vegetable stock if you prefer)
1 tablespoon olive oil
1 tablespoon chopped fresh mint leaves (lime mint works well
    if you have any)
Coconut cream (optional)
salt and freshly ground black pepper

Put the lentils in a bowl, cover with cold water and leave overnight. Next day drain and rinse them with fresh water. In a large saucepan, sauté the onion in the olive oil for 2–3 minutes until it colours, add the garlic and spices and cook for 1–2 minutes. Add the lentils and tomato purée and stir well before adding the bouillon or stock. Bring to the boil and simmer for about 20 minutes. Add the chopped mint and continue to simmer until the lentils are soft (about 10 minutes). Purée with a stick blender. Check the seasoning adding more mint if need be and serve hot with a little coconut cream twirled on top of each bowl (optional).

Spiced vegetable noodles

- ½ tablespoon grated fresh ginger root or use galangal root if you have it.
- ½ tablespoon grated fresh turmeric root
- 4–6 shiitake mushrooms, sliced (used fresh or soak in hot water before use if dried)
- 1–2 courgettes cut into thin batons
- 1–2 carrots cut into very thin batons or julienned in a food processor
- 1–2 spring onions sliced into strips.
- 1 handful of sprouted mung beans or green lentils
- 1 red or yellow pepper, deseeded and finely sliced
- 6oz/175g fine rice noodles (you can add more if you want)
- 2 tablespoons light soy sauce
- 2 tablespoons Thai fish sauce
- 2 tablespoons rice wine (or sherry)
- 2 tablespoons groundnut oil

Heat the wok and then add the groundnut oil. Stir fry the ginger, turmeric and mushrooms for 2–3 minutes, then add the courgettes and carrots and stir fry for 3–4 minutes. Add the noodles and toss well with the vegetables for 1–2 minutes then add the soy sauce, fish sauce and rice wine (or sherry) and the sliced spring onions. Stir gently together for 1–2 minutes and serve. Optionally, you can add strips of cooked chicken or ham hock with the vegetables or stir in some cooked brown shrimps when you add the sliced spring onions.

Mrs Daya's chicken curry[6]

1–2 tablespoons olive oil (enough to cover the pan)
1 medium chicken, skinned and jointed
1 large onion, very finely sliced
8 tomatoes, skinned, deseeded and finely diced
8 small potatoes, peeled
3 cardamom pods
3 pieces cinnamon bark (about 1–2inches long)
3 cloves
10 whole black peppers
2 teaspoons ginger, finely chopped
1½ teaspoons garlic, finely chopped or crushed
¾ teaspoon ground cayenne
¾ teaspoon ground turmeric
1 teaspoon ground coriander
2 teaspoons tomato purée
Salt to taste
½ teaspoon *garam masala*
A couple of handfuls of fresh coriander
approx. 3 tablespoons olive oil

Cover the bottom of a large saucepan with olive oil and heat.
Add the cloves, cardamom, pepper, cinnamon and fry for a
couple of minutes to release the flavour of the spices.

Add the onions and cook until softened and golden – do
not let them brown. Add the tomatoes, garlic, ginger, cayenne,
turmeric, tomato purée and salt. Stir regularly while cooking
to ensure that the mixture does not stick or start to burn. The
sauce (*masala*) is cooked once the oil separates and the colour
darkens, approx. 15–20 minutes.

Add the potatoes and cook for about 10 minutes. Add the
chicken, coat the pieces in sauce and cook for a few minutes

until golden. Add just enough hot water to cover. Stir and simmer until cooked. (about 5–10 minutes). Check that the chicken pieces are cooked through but do not let the potatoes get too soft .

Add *garam masala* and fresh coriander and serve with Mrs Daya's rice.

Mrs Daya's rice

    1½ cups of basmati rice
    6 cups of water
    1 teaspoon salt
    2 pieces cinnamon bark (about 1–2inches long)
    2 cloves
    3 black peppercorns
    3 cardamom pods

Rinse the rice twice in very hot water and then leave to sit in hot water for at least 15 mins

Heat the water in a large saucepan with the salt, cardamom, cinnamon, cloves and peppercorns. When the water is boiling, add the rice and turn down the heat to a rolling boiling for about 10 minutes until the rice is just cooked. Cooking time depends on the age of the rice – it may need a little longer.

Drain excess water from the rice, return to the stove (heat off) and cover for 20 mins to allow the rice to absorb any remaining water. Rice grains should be separate and fluffy. Serve with Mrs Daya's chicken curry.

Mrs Daya's vegetable curry

1–2 tablespoons of olive oil (enough to cover the pan)
1 teaspoon fenugreek
1 teaspoon mustard seeds
1 medium onion, finely sliced
8 tomatoes, skinned, deseeded and finely diced
6 medium new potatoes (e.g. Charlotte or Exquisa), peeled and parboiled
1 aubergine, chopped into 1inch cubes and placed in a bowl of cold water to prevent discoloration
1 cup of frozen peas
1 cup of French beans, washed and cut in half
1 heaped teaspoon garlic, finely chopped or crushed
2 heaped teaspoons, ginger, finely chopped
1 teaspoon turmeric
¾ teaspoon salt
1 teaspoon tomato purée
1 tablespoon chopped coriander leaves to garnish

Heat the oil over a gently heat in a large saucepan. Add the fenugreek and mustard seeds and fry gently for a minute or so. Add the onions and cook until softened and golden – do not let them brown. Add the tomatoes, ginger, garlic, turmeric and salt and stir.

Cook on a medium heat until the oil starts to separate and the mixture (*masala*) darkens, approx. 20 minutes. Watch closely, stir every few minutes and be careful not to let it burn. In the meantime, cook the beans and peas in boiling water for 2–3 minutes and set aside.

When the *masala* is ready, add the parboiled potatoes, stir and cook for another 2 minutes. Add the peas and green beans.

Squeeze out excess water from aubergine pieces and add to

the saucepan. Stir well. Continue to cook on a medium heat for about 20 minutes, until the aubergine is soft and has turned slightly green. Place in a dish and sprinkle with coriander.

Serve with Mrs Daya's rice or chapatti and salad with some mango chutney.

Potent curry herbs

(See Appendix 1 or Glossary for explanation of any Ayurvedic terms)

While turmeric seems to dominate discussion of the herbs and spices used in curry other regular ingredients are also therapeutic.

Cardamom *(Elettaria cardamomum)* – appetite stimulant, carminative, diaphoretic, expectorant, stomachic. Used in Ayurveda for colds, coughs, indigestion, loss of appetite and regarded as clearing *kapha* from the stomach and lungs and stimulating *agni*.

Cayenne *(Capsicum annuum)* – circulatory stimulant, warming, diaphoretic, antiseptic, antispasmodic, carminative. Used in Ayurveda as a strong stimulant and to dispel both internal and external cold and nurture *agni*. Excess can aggravate inflammatory conditions and *pitta*. It is considered as *rajasic* so potentially irritant.

Cinnamon *(Cinnamomum verum)*; Chinese cinnamon is C. *cassia* – stimulant, diaphoretic, carminative, expectorant, diuretic, anti-oxidant, analgesic, warming, haemostatic, antiseptic, vermifuge, anti-microbial, antispasmodic. Used in Ayurveda for strengthening and harmonising the circulation, strengthening the heart, warming the kidneys and encouraging *agni*.

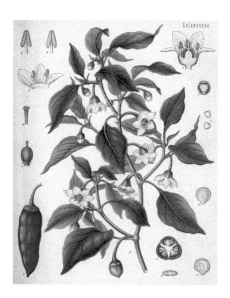

Cayenne (*Capsicum annuum*) from
Franz Eugen Köhler (1897) *Köhler's Medizinal-Pflanzen*

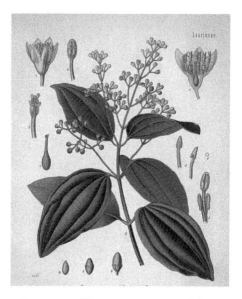

Cinnamon (*Cinnamomum verum*) from
Franz Eugen Köhler (1897) *Köhler's Medizinal-Pflanzen*

Clove (*Syzygium aromaticum*) – mild local anaesthetic, carminative, expectorant, warming, stimulant, antiseptic, anti-histamine, antispasmodic, anti-oxidant, aphrodisiac. Used in Ayurveda to dispel chills, stimulate the lungs and stomach, heating, energising and *rajasic*.

Coriander (*Coriandrum sativum*) – stimulant, carminative, anti-oxidant, diaphoretic. Japanese research in 2001 suggested it may chelate lead and possibly other heavy metals[7]. Used in Ayurveda for *pitta* disorders especially those involving the digestive tract and urinary system,

Cumin (*Cuminum cyminum*) – carminative, anti-spasmodic, anti-oxidant, stimulant, aphrodisiac, diuretic, emmenagogue. Used in Ayurveda for indigestion, diarrhoea, dysentery and to counter hot, pungent foods.

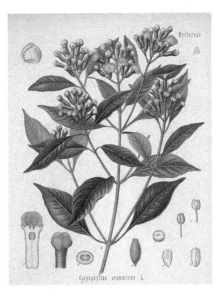

Clove (*Syzygium aromaticum*) from
Franz Eugen Köhler (1897) *Köhler's Medizinal-Pflanzen*

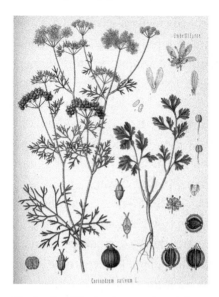

Coriander (*Coriandrum sativum*) from
Franz Eugen Köhler (1897) *Köhler's Medizinal-Pflanzen*

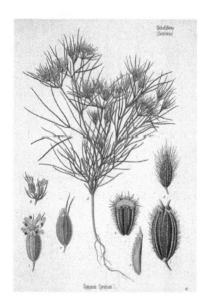

Cumin (*Cuminum cyminum*) from
Franz Eugen Köhler (1897) *Köhler's Medizinal-Pflanzen*

Fenugreek *(Trigonella foenum-graecum)* – stimulant, tonic, expectorant, aphrodisiac, demulcent, emollient, nutrient, anti-inflammatory, diuretic, hypoglycaemic, galactagogue, oxytocic. Used in Ayurveda as a strengthening food in debility, to strengthen and soothe the digestive tract, and encourage milk flow. The seeds are generally used but the aerial stems and leaves are taken in both China and the Middle East for dysentery and menstrual period cramps.

Galangal *(Alpinia officinarum)* – carminative, stomachic, stimulant, diaphoretic, anti-fungal, anti-rheumatic. Used in Ayurveda to stimulate *pitta* and help clear excess *vata* and *kapha*. Hildegard of Bingen (1098–1179) recommended it for angina pectoris.

Ginger *(Zingiber officinale)* – anti-inflammatory, carminative, antispasmodic, expectorant, vasodilator, anti-cholesterol, circulatory stimulant, anti-emetic, anti-oxidant, diaphoretic. Regarded in Ayurveda as the most *sattvic* of the spices and *vishwabhesaj* – "the universal medicine". Taken with honey to relieve *kapha*, with rock salt to relieve *pitta* and with *misri* (rock sugar) to relieve *pitta*. Used to stimulate *agni*. Dry ginger will reduce *kapha* and fresh ginger for deranged *vata*.

Pepper *(Piper nigrum)* – stimulant, expectorant, carminative, febrifuge, anthelmintic. Used in Ayurveda as a powerful digestive stimulant to burn *ama* and energise *agni*. Mixed with ghee it is used topically as a nasal decongestant and to heal skin inflammations and with honey as an expectorant. it is a good antidote to excessive intake of cold or raw foods and is *rajasic* in character.

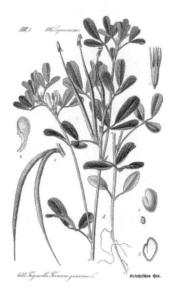

Fenugreek (*Trigonella foenum-graecum*) from
Prof. Dr. Otto Wilhelm Thomé (1885) *Flora von Deutschland,
Österreich und der Schweiz.*

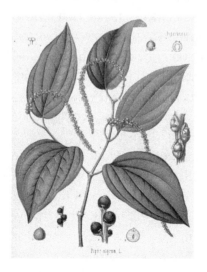

Pepper (*Piper nigrum*) from Franz Eugen Köhler (1897)
Köhler's Medizinal-Pflanzen.

Chapter 8

Turmeric for all

In May 1995 the US Patent Office granted the University of
Mississippi Medical Center a patent for "Use of Turmeric in
Wound Healing". Patents mean that someone, somewhere
"owns" something and others have to pay for the privilege of
using the invention or be in breach of the law. But, sprinkling
a pinch of turmeric onto their children's cuts and grazes was
something Indian mothers had been doing for generations – so
how could such a long-standing activity suddenly be "owned"
by the University of Mississippi?

The patent was challenged by India's Council of Scientific
and Industrial Research, which was able to easily demonstrate that turmeric had been used in India for centuries for
wound healing and a great many other things: the Mississippi
researchers' claim for a "novel invention" was no such thing.
Eventually the patent was annulled. It was the first time a
patent based on the traditional knowledge of a developing
country had been successfully challenged.

So, if the supplement producers couldn't patent turmeric, they turned their attention to the next best thing: the group of chemicals that help differentiate turmeric from other members of the *Curcuma* spp. – the curcuminoids responsible for the rich yellow colour. You can't patent a single chemical only a unique application, invention or process, which means that the hundreds of patents relating to curcumin have all involved some novel aspect of extraction, formulation, or use. There are patents using curcumin for "formula feed for adult butterfishes", for "ink composition", for making "instant spicy white prawn" or for a "fast-dissolving soil-drip-irrigation fertilizer for greenhouse crops" – as well as a great many for improving bioavailability or treating specific health problems.

Having patented the product, the next stage is to turn it to financial advantage, hence the current plethora of curcumin marketing messages and promotional activity aimed at persuading consumers that one particular extract is better than another – and that both are far superior to the ordinary turmeric that has been used for centuries. Supporting these claims are a number of small scale clinical trials which, as already discussed, often involve very few patients, are generally of short duration and are rarely controlled (i.e. compared with placebo) or "double-blind (i.e. neither researchers nor patients knows who is given placebo and who is given the test remedy to avoid bias in the results). As critical researchers have concluded: "... the beneficial effects of curcumin and derivatives demonstrated *in vitro* have not been adequately confirmed by randomized, double-blind, placebo-controlled clinical trials, as well as the potential occurrence of harmful side-effects resulting from herb–drug interaction, does not justify a wide and uncontrolled use of curcumin in therapy"[1].

This is not to suggest that the various curcumin products on the market are not effective or their claims are entirely without substance: these products have brought relief to many people suffering from arthritic problems, digestive disorders, depression, skin complaints and much more. What we don't have – because there is no benefit to be gained by spending a great deal of money on clinical trials using a whole plant that cannot be patented – is the scientific evidence to demonstrate that taking turmeric could be just as effective.

As discussed at the start of this book, an in-depth review of curcumin chemistry published in January 2017, raised a number of questions about the possible efficacy of the chemical owing to its instability. While this triggered several media reports critical of curcumin, it did not encourage the numerous online bloggers and healthy living websites to question the various claims made for different curcumin extracts.

Also, as discussed earlier, over the years there have been a few studies exploring the therapeutic properties of some of the other secondary metabolites found in turmeric as well as the break-down products formed when curcumin is digested. One concluded that "our findings strongly suggested that the degradation products should make important contributions to the diverse biological activities of curcumin"[2]. In other words, the fact that it is broken down in the digestive process really doesn't matter because the resulting chemicals might be just as therapeutically effective. It suggested that the emphasis on and preoccupation with curcumin bioavailability may have been a complete red herring. Others are equally sceptical: "It is very important and ethically relevant to not provide people with ambiguous information about the benefit coming from the use of curcumin in chronic inflammatory diseases and to focus the attention on the 'risk to benefit' ratio of supplemental therapy with curcumin, which might be shifted towards the 'risk'."[1]

Turmeric is undoubtedly a very valuable herb which has only started to be fully appreciated in the West in the past decade, while curcumin research has highlighted a variety of new applications in addition to its many traditional uses. At the same time, the EU's Traditional Herbal Medicinal Products directive limits the range of actions that suppliers of turmeric capsules can claim for their products, should they wish to apply for a licence under the directive. It relegates turmeric – and also curcumin – to be "food supplements": unlicensed products that cannot make any medicinal claims. Curcumin supplement producers tend to eulogise on their packaging about their bio-availability, but cannot suggest on that packaging for which ailments this particular extract may be especially effective.

As a result would-be users of curcumin or turmeric supplements must search the Internet – or their herbals – for information. Only the most recent western herbals devote much attention to turmeric or recommend it for anything other than arthritis, skin problems or digestive disorders, while not all Internet information sources are entirely unbiased and much may be anecdotal.

While most of the clinical trials to date involving curcumin, or occasionally turmeric, have been inconclusive, in their review, Kunnumakkara et al.[3] list many more that are still underway: many take years to complete and report their findings, some never do. One currently still recruiting, for example, is looking at a combination of using curcumin and yoga therapy for those at risk of Alzheimer's disease. It was first announced in March 2013, is still recruiting participants and expects to report findings by December 2018[4]. Many others operate in similarly protracted timescales.

With pharmaceutical drugs, early small scale clinical trials and safety studies are generally followed by much larger, multi-national trials which can continue for years; it can take decades before a new drug is finally approved as safe and efficacious. That isn't going to happen for either turmeric or curcumin for the basic economic fact that the expense is unlikely ever to be justified by the likely return – and if anyone did prove that turmeric really was "nature's miracle" a great many people would simply continue to drink daily glasses of golden milk using culinary grade turmeric rather than buy expensive capsules.

Turmeric "food supplement" capsules may provide some assurance that they contain only turmeric and no "fillers", as manufacturers are required to meet certain quality control standards. Buying culinary turmeric does carry the risk of unwanted additives coloured with lead chromate or other nasties or you can play safe and follow the advice from *The Times of India*[5] mentioned earlier and buy whole rhizomes. However you choose to take it, turmeric is likely to deliver benefits for a wide spectrum of ailments: not so much a miracle, but just another of nature's wonderful herbal medicines waiting to be discovered.

> "Herbs are gathered together in an apothecary's shop ... there is in the world a natural order of apothecary's shops for all the fields and meadows, all the mountains and hills are such shops. All nature is like one single apothecary's shop, covered only with the roof of heaven ..."
>
> Paracelsus (1493–1541)[6]

Appendix 1

Ayurvedic approach to food and herbs

The term Ayurveda comes from two Indian words: *ayur*, "life", and *veda*, "knowledge", Ayurvedic medicine is thus sometimes described as a "knowledge of how to live". It teaches that good health is the responsibility of the individual with illness seen in terms of imbalance, while herbs and dietary controls are used to restore equilibrium.

As with traditional western Graeco-Roman or Galenic medicine Ayurveda sees the world and everything in it as composed of basic elements: earth, air, fire and water, just as in the Graeco-Roman model, but with the addition of a fifth element, aether. These universal elements are converted by the digestive fire (*agni*) into three humours (*tri doshas*) which influence individual health and temperament. Air and aether yield *vata* (wind), fire produces the humour *pitta* (fire or bile) while earth and water combine to give *kapha* (phlegm). The waste products of digestion are *ama* and if digestion is weak then *ama* accumulates and may lead to illness, so a key dietary aim is to support *agni*.

The humours must remain well balanced as any excess or deficit can lead to illness. Food and herbs are classified as tending to increase or damage the humours so an excessive amount of one type of food can lead to imbalance. Too many sweet carbohydrates, for example, increases *kapha* and excess here may cause such problems as catarrh, oedema or water retention.

Kapha is cold, wet, slow and heavy, so is balanced by a diet of warm, light and dry foods and hot, bitter herbs such as cinnamon, pepper and turmeric.

Pitta is hot, light, soft and clear and an imbalance may be associated with inflammatory and infectious conditions, boils, sores and feverish illnesses. It is treated with purgatives and light, cooling remedies such as grapes, liquorice, and sugar.

Vata is the most powerful of the *doshas* and is light, dry, cool and mobile. Imbalance here leads to dryness, insomnia, arthritis, rheumatism, fatigue and constipation. Sweet, sour and salty foods will reduce *vata* while pungent herbs, tonics and demulcents, such as psyllium seeds, can help stimulate it.

Ayurveda also envisions two fundamental principles: *purusha* – the primal spirit and *prakruti* – nature or primal matter. *Prakruti* consists of three *gunas*: *sattva* – the principle of light, intelligence and harmony; *rajas* – energy, activity, emotion and turbulence and *tamas* – inertia, darkness, and dullness. Herbs and foods also contain the characteristics of the *gunas* so can also increase or reduce these attributes.

Herbs and foods are also classified by taste and these must also be kept in balance for good health. In Ayurveda, the tastes are defined as: sweet, sour, salty, astringent, pungent and bitter. Traditionally all six tastes should be present at each meal to ensure balance, so it could contain, for example, foods and herbs such as:

Table 3: Examples of Ayurvedic tastes balancing a meal

Taste	Food	Herb/Spice/Flavouring
Sweet	Mango	Fennel
Sour	Yoghurt	Lime juice
Salty	Celery	Seaweed
Astringent	Chicken	Pomegranate seeds
Pungent	Onion	Cardamom
Bitter	Aubergine	Turmeric

There is obviously a great deal more to Ayurveda than this very brief summary and some useful sources are listed in Notes and References[1].

Appendix 2

Traditional Chinese Medicine (TCM)

Traditional Chinese medical theory is also based on elements, this time wood, fire, earth, metal, and water. Each of these five elements is linked to a long list of attributes which include bodily organs and functions, the seasons, foods, tastes, sounds, emotions and much more. As in Galenic and Ayurvedic medicine, good health involves keeping these attributes in balance. The elements also influence each other in a seasonal cycle – thus winter rains give rise to spring growth (wood) which leads to summer fires, then ashes (earth) from which comes metal on which water condenses. If any element – and its related organs, emotions, bodily functions etc – is weak then the next element in the cycle will also be weak.

Chinese five element theory dates back around 5,000 years – long before our current understanding of anatomy and physiology and the five "solid" and five "hollow" organs it identifies bear little relation to modern scientific understanding. To

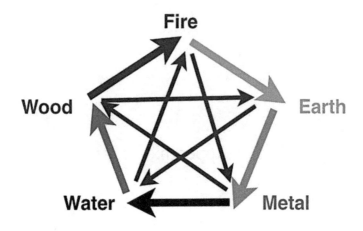

Chinese five element model showing some of the
influences between the elements.

differentiate these organ "concepts" from today's anatomical
understanding, they are generally written with capital letters.

Table 4: Some five element associations

	Wood	Fire	Earth	Metal	Water
Season	Spring	Summer	Late summer	Autumn	Winter
Solid organ	Liver	Heart	Spleen	Lung	Kidney
Hollow organ	Gallbladder	Small Intestine	Stomach	Large intestine	Urinary bladder
Sense organs	Eyes	Tongue	Mouth	Nose	Ears
Taste	Sour	Bitter	Sweet	Pungent/Acrid	Salty
Tissues	Tendons	Blood vessels	Muscles	Skin	Bone

TCM also recognises five "fundamental substances" which
can be translated as vital energy (*qì*), Blood (*xue*), vital
essence (*jīng*), body fluids (*jin-ye*) and spirit (*shèn*). These substances flow through the body and any obstruction to their

movements, excess or deficiency can lead to imbalance and ill health. Both vital energy and Blood can be obstructed in their flow and stagnate, which is seen as a cause of various types of pain. Acupuncture and herbal remedies may be used to normalise flow.

Chinese theory also talks of both internal and external causes of disease. Internal causes are largely linked to emotions (joy, anger, sadness, worry, fear, grief, and shock) while external causes are wind, cold, heat, dampness, dryness and fire. These external causes can initially affect the exterior, but also move inwards into the body.

Herbs are used to treat these various causes and turmeric (*jiang huang*) and other *Curcuma*, spp. are variously used to move *qì*, clear Blood stagnation or expel wind.

To this is added the concept of *yin* and *yang* – *yin* being inward, dark, passive while *yang* is outward, light and active. *Yin* and *yang* are both present in all things and, again, must be kept in balance to prevent disease. There is obviously a great deal more to traditional Chinese medicine than this very brief summary and some useful sources are listed in Notes and References[2].

Appendix 3

Making turmeric cream or ointment

1. Turmeric ointment

You will need ground or fresh turmeric rhizome, cold pressed sun-flower oil, cocoa butter and beeswax.

- Heat 20g of ground turmeric or chopped fresh turmeric rhizome in 200ml of cold pressed sunflower oil in a double saucepan or bain marie over water for at least 90 minutes. Do not allow the oil to boil and check the water in the lower pan regularly to avoid it boiling dry. Strain the oil mixture through muslin or a fine sieve.
- In a clean double saucepan or bain marie over water melt 10g or beeswax and 20g of cocoa butter. When melted add 120ml of the strained oil. Continue to heat for a few seconds to ensure all is dissolved (cooler oil may re-solidify the wax and butter).

- Pour the hot mixture into clean ointment pots and allow to cool. You will need two 60ml pots or similar.

2. Turmeric cream

You will need ground or fresh turmeric rhizome, emulsifying flakes (lanette wax), soft paraffin, sunflower oil, glycerine, and water.

- Make an emulsifying ointment by melting together 30g emulsifying flakes, 50g of soft paraffin and 20ml of sunflower oil, in a double saucepan or bain marie over water.
- When melted add 30g of ground turmeric or chopped fresh turmeric rhizome and 110ml each of water and glycerine.
- Heat the mixture for at least 90 minutes in the double saucepan. Do not allow it to boil and check the water in the lower pan regularly to avoid it boiling dry.
- Squeeze the mixture through muslin into a clean basin as quickly as possible while it is still hot (wear rubber gloves). Stir the mixture continually as it cools and thickens to avoid the cream from separating.
- Once cool and set store in small pots. You will need enough pots for about 200–250ml of cream, depending how much you have managed to squeeze out.

Notes and references

Chapter 1; Fashionable hype ... and confusion

1. Curcumin Resource Database (CRDB) http://www.crdb.in/index.php
2. Nelson, K. M., Dahlin, J. L., Bisson, J., Graham, J., Pauli, G. F., and Walters, M. A.(2017): "The essential medical chemistry of curcumin", *Journal of Medicinal Chemistry,* **60**, 1620–1637.
3. http://www.turmericsave.co.uk
4. http://purelyholistic.org/product/turmeric-curcumin-bioperine
5. https://www.webmd.com/vitamins-supplements/ingredientmono-662-TURMERIC.aspx?activeIngredientId=662&activeIngredientName=TURMERIC&source=3
6. Nagaraja, T.N., and Desiraju, T. (1993) "Effects of chronic consumption of metanil yellow by developing and adult rats on brain regional levels of noradrenaline, dopamine and serotonin, on acetylcholine esterase activity and on operant conditioning", *Food and Chemical Toxicology,* **31(1)**, 41–44.
7. https://www.fda.gov/safety/recalls/ucm515328.htm
8. https://www.turmericforhealth.com/general-info/how-to-test-turmeric-powder-for-quality-and-avoid-adulterated-products
9. Rhizoma Curcuma longa in *WHO Monographs on Selected Medicinal Plants* – Vol. 1 http://apps.who.int/medicinedocs/en/d/Js2200e/14.html

10. Mancuso, C., and Barone, E. (2009) "Curcumin in clinical practice: myth or reality?" *Trends in Pharmacological Sciences*, 30, 333–334.

Chapter 2: Meet the plant and its traditional uses

1. Trease, G. E., and Evans, W. C. (1983) *Pharmacognosy*, 12th edition, Ballière Tindall, London.
2. http://powo.science.kew.org/taxon/urn:lsid:ipni.org:names:796451-1
3. Huttin, W. (1998) *Tropical Herbs and Spices of Thailand*, Asia Books, Bangkok.
4. Li, S., Yuan, W., Deng, G., Wang, P., Yang, P., and Aggarwal, B. B. (2011) "Chemical composition and product quality control or turmeric (*Curcuma longa*)", *Pharmaceutical Crops*, 2, 28–54.
5. Singh, S., Sankar, B., Rajesh, S., Sahoo, K., Subudhi, E., and Nayak, S.(2011) "Chemical composition of turmeric oil (*Curcuma longa L*. cv. Roma) and its antimicrobial activity against eye infecting pathogens", *Journal of Essential Oil Research*, 23:6, 11–18.
6. Ravindra, P. N., Nirmal Babu, K., and Sivaraman, K. eds. (2007) *Turmeric: The Genus Curcuma*, CRC Press, Boca Raton, Florida, pp.10–11.
7. Jain, S.K., and DeFilippo, R. A. (1991) *Medicinal Plants of India*, Reference Publications, Algonac, Michigan.
8. Leon, C., and Yu-Lin, L. (2017) *Chinese Medicinal Plants, Herbal Drugs and Substitutes: an identification guide*, Kew Publishing, London.
9. Prasad, S., and Aggarwak, N. B. (2011) "Turmeric, the Golden Spice", Chapter 13 in *Herbal Medicine: Biomolecular and Clinical Aspects*. 2nd edition. Eds. Benzie, I. F. F., and Wachtel-Galor, S., CRC Press/Taylor & Francis, Boca Raton, Florida.
10. Bhishagratna, K. K. L. (1907) *An English Translation of The Shushruta Samhita*, Vol. 1, pp. 347–360, Calcutta, reprinted 2015, www.forgottenbooks.com.
11. Lad, U., and Lad, V. (1994) *Ayurvedic Cooking for Self-Healing*, Ayurvedic Press, Albuquerque, New Mexico.
12. Jain, S.K., and DeFilippo, R. A. (1991) *Medicinal Plants of India*, Reference Publications, Algonac, Michigan, quoting Bodding, P. O. (1927) "Studies in Sanmtal medicine and connected folklore II. Santam medicine:" *Memoirs of the Asiatic Society of Bengal*, 10, 133–426.

13. Frawley, D. and Lad, V. (1988) *The Yoga of Herbs*, Lotus Press, Santa Fe, New Mexico.

14. Bensky, D. and Gamble, A. (1986) *Chinese Herbal Medicine*, Eastland Press, Seattle.

15. Yang, L. (1784) *Shanghan wenyi tiaobian (Systematic Differentiation of Cold Damage and Warm Epidemics)*, reprinted Xueyuan Chubanshe, Beijing, 2006.

16. Blalack, J. (2012) "An everyday warm disease formula: Ascending and Descending Powder (*Sheng Jiang San*)", *Journal of Chinese Medicine*, **98**, 18–23.

17. Grieve, M. (1931) *A Modern Herbal*, Jonathan Cape, London. p.822–823.

18. Mills, S., and Bone, K. (2000) *Principles and Practice of Phytotherapy*, Churchill Livingstone, London. p.569.

19. Bone, K., and Mills, S. (2013) *Principles and Practice of Phytotherapy*, 2nd edition Churchill Livingstone, London. p.900.

20. Wren, R. C. (1988) *Potter's New Cyclopaedia of Botanical Drugs and Preparations* (revised by Williamson, A. M., and Evans, F. J.) C .W. Daniel, Saffron Walden.

21. Bartram, T. (1995) *Encyclopaedia of Herbal Medicine*, Grace Publishers, Christchurch, Dorset.

Chapter 3: Focussing on the curcuminoids

1. Curcumin Resource Database http://www.crdb.in

2. Priyadarsini, K. I. (2014) "The chemistry of curcumin: from extraction to therapeutic agent", *Molecules*, **19**, 20091–20112.

3. Sakey, R., Bafubiandi-Mulaba, A.F., Rajnikanth, V., Varaprasad, K., Reddy, N.N., and Raju, K.M. (2012) "Development and characterization of curcumin loaded silver nanoparticle hydrogels for antibacterial and drug delivery applications", *Journal of Inorganic and Organometallic Polymers and Materials*, **22**, 1254–1262.

4. "Indian police impound synthetic curcumin." http://www.sabinsa. com/newsroom/press-releases/pr20150625.html

5. "Recall of food supplements Miradin and Fortodol due to presence of unauthorised substance (nimesulide)." http://webarchive. nationalarchives.gov.uk/20111206062936/http://www.food.gov.uk/ enforcement/alerts/2009/mar/miradinfortodol

6. Nelson, K. M., Dahlin, J. L., Bisson, J., Graham, J., Pauli, G. F., and Walters, M. A.(2017): "The essential medical chemistry of curcumin", *Journal of Medicinal Chemistry*, **60**, 1620–1637.

7. Baker, M. (2017) "Deceptive curcumin offers cautionary tale for chemists", *Nature*, **11** January 2017, https://www.nature.com/news/deceptive-curcumin-offers-cautionary-tale-for-chemists-1.21269

8. Wahlström, B., and Blennow, G. (1978) "A study on the fate of curcumin in the rat", *Acta Pharmacologica et Toxicologica (Copenhagen)*, **43:2**, 259–265.

9. Lin, J. K., Pan, M. H, and Lin-Shiau, S.Y. (2000) "Recent studies on the biofunctions and biotransformations of curcumin", *BioFactors*, **13(1–4)**, 153–158. Phase II metabolites include curcumin glucuronide, duhydrocurcumin glucuronide, tetrahydrocurcumin glycuronide and tetrahydrocurcumin.

10. Osawa, T. (2007) "Nephroprotective and hepatoprotective effects of curcuminoids", *Advances in Experimental Medicine and Biology*, **595**, 407–423.

11. Dutta, B. (2015) "Study of secondary metabolite constituents and curcumin contents of six different species of genus *Curcuma*", *Journal of Medicinal Plant Studies*, **3(5)** 116–119.

12. Singh, S., Sankar, B., Rajesh, S., Sahoo, K., Subudhi, E., and Nayak, S.(2011) "Chemical composition of turmeric oil (*Curcuma longa L.* cv. Roma) and its antimicrobial activity against eye infecting pathogens", *Journal of Essential Oil Research*, **23:6**, 11–18; Jayaprakasha, G.K., Negi, P. S., Anandharamakrishnan, C., and Sakariah K.K. (2001) "Chemical composition of turmeric oil–a byproduct from turmeric oleoresin industry and its inhibitory activity against different fungi", *Zeitschrift für Naturforschung C.*, **56(1–2)**, 40–44.

13. Cuomo, J., Appendino, G., Dern, A. S., Schneider, E., McKinnon, T.P., Brown, M.J., Togni, S., and Dixon, B. M., (2011) "Comparative absorption of a standardized curcuminoid mixture and its lecithin formulation", *Journal of Natural Products*, **74(4)**, 664–669.

14. The authors of this particular study included scientists working for Usana Health Sciences – a maker of complex nutritional supplements.

Chapter 4: Extracts and supplements

1. http://www.crdb.in/patent.php
2. Shoba, G., Joy, D., Joseph, T., Majeed, M., Rajendran, R., and Srinivas, P. S. S. R. (1997) "Influence of piperine on the pharmacokinetics of curcumin in animals and human volunteers", *Planta Medica*, **64(4)**, 353–356.
3. Bishnoi, M., Chopra, K., Rongzhu, L., and Kulkarni, S. K. (2011) "Protective effect of curcumin and its combination with piperine (bioavailability enhancer) against haloperidol-associated neurotoxicity: cellular and neurochemical evidence", *Neurotoxicity Research*, **20:3**, 215–225.
4. http://www.thrivibrant.com/the-truth-about-bcm-95-vs-curcumin-95-vs-meriva/
5. Cox, K. H., Pipingas, A., and Scholey, A. S. B., (2015) "Investigation of the effects of solid lipid curcumin on cognition and mood in a healthy older population", *Journal of Psychopharmacology*, **29(5)**, 642–651.
6. Cuomo. J., Appendino, G., Dern, A. S., Schneider, E., McKinnon, T. P., Brown, M. J., Togni, S., and Dixon, B. M. (2011) "Comparative absorption of a standardized curcuminoid mixture and its lecithin formulation", *Journal of Natural Products*, **74(4)**, 664–669.
7. http://theravalues.com/english/research-clinical-trials/
8. https://data.integrativepro.com/product-literature/info/theracurmin-info-sheet.pdf
9. Naz, S., Ilyas, S., Paeveen, Z., and Javed, S. (2010) "Chemical analysis of essential oils from turmeric (*Curcuma longa*) rhizome through GC-MS", *Asian Journal of Chemistry*, **22(4)**, 3153–3158.
10. Lopresti, A., and Drummond, P. (2017) "Efficacy of curcumin, and a saffron/curcumin combination for the treatment of major depression: A randomised, double-blind, placebo-controlled study", *Journal of Affective Disorders*, **207**, 188–196.
11. Patent: "A water soluble composition comprising curcumin having enhanced bioavailability and process thereof" http://www.crdb.in/patdetails.php?id=515
12. Jäger, R., Lowery, R. P., Calvanese, A. V., Joy, J. M., Purpura, M., and Wilson, J. M. (2014) "Comparative absorption of curcumin

formulations". *Nutrition Journal,* **13:11**, published online 24 January 2014, https://doi.org/10.1186/1475-2891-13-11.

13. http://omniactives.com/press-releases/ultrasol-curcumin-lin e-curcuwin-granted-patent-for-sports-performance-benefits

14. Purpura, M., Lowery, R. P., Wilson, J. M., Mannan, H., Münch, G., and Razmovski-Naumovski, V. (2017) "Analysis of different innovative formulations of curcumin for improved relative oral bioavailability in human subjects", *European Journal of Nutrition,* published online 16 February 2017. https://doi.org/10.1007/s00394-016-1376-9.

15. http://www.naturex.com/Media2/Press-releases/Vitafoods-Europ e-2017-New-natural-solutions-target-healthy-ageing

16. https://www.alibaba.com/showroom/price-curcumin.html

17. Panel on Food Additives and Nutrient Sources added to Food (2010) "Re-evaluation of curcumin (E100) as a food additive", *European Food Safety Authority Journal.,* **8(9)**, 1679 [46 pp.].

18. Abdel-Tawab, M., Werz, O., and Schubert-Zsilavecz, M. (2011) "*Boswellia serrata*: An overall assessment of *in vitro*, preclinical, pharmacokinetic and clinical data", *Clinical Pharmacokinetics,* **50 (6)**, 349–369.

Chapter 5: Curcumin vs turmeric

1. Singh, S., Sankar, B., Rajesh, S., Sahoo, K., Subudhi, E., and Nayak, S.(2011) "Chemical composition of turmeric oil (*Curcuma longa* L. cv. Roma) and its antimicrobial activity against eye infecting pathogens", *Journal of Essential Oil Research,* **23:6**, 11–18; Jayaprakasha, G.K., Negi, P. S., Anandharamakrishnan, C., and Sakariah K.K. (2001) "Chemical composition of turmeric oil–a byproduct from turmeric oleoresin industry and its inhibitory activity against different fungi", *Zeitschrift für Naturforschung C.,* **56(1–2)**, 40–44.

2. Chandra, D., and Gupta, S. S. (1972) "Anti-inflammatory and anti-arthritic activity of volatile oil of *Curcuma longa (Haldi)*", *Indian Journal of Medical Research,* **60**, 138–142.

3. Nelson, K. M., Dahlin, J. L., Bisson, J., Graham, J., Pauli, G. F., and Walters, M. A. (2017): "The essential medical chemistry of curcumin", *Journal of Medicinal Chemistry,* **60**, 1620–1637.

4. Baker, M. (2017) "Deceptive curcumin offers cautionary tale for chemists", *Nature*, 11 January 2017, http://www.nature.com/news/deceptive-curcumin-offers-cautionary-tale-for-chemists-1.21269

5. Wahlström, B., and Blennow, G. (1978) "A study on the fate of curcumin in the rat", *Acta Pharmacologica et Toxicologica (Copenhagen)*, **43:2**, 259–265.

6. Bone, K., and Mills, S. (2013) *Principles and Practice of Phytotherapy*, 2nd edn, Churchill Livingstone Elsevier, p.901.

7. The German Commission E is a scientific advisory board of the "Bundesinstitut für Arzneimittel und Medizinprodukte" (the German equivalent of the UK's Medicines and Healthcare Products Regulatory Agency (MHRA) or the Food and Drug Administration in the USA, It was formed in 1978 and publishes basic monographs on many medicinal herbs. An English version of the monographs can be accessed at http://cms.herbalgram.org/commissione/

8. Kuroda, M., Mimaki Y., Nishiyama, T., Mae, T., Kishida, H., Tsukagawa, M., Takahashi, K., Kawada, T., Nakagawa, K., and Kitahara, M. (2005) " Hypoglycemic effects of turmeric (*Curcuma longa* L. rhizomes) on genetically diabetic KK-A mice", *Biological and Pharmaceurical Bullerin*, **28(5)**, 937–939.

9. Tang, M., Larson-Meyer, D. E., and Liebman, M. (2008) "Effect of cinnamon and turmeric on urinary oxalate excretion, plasma lipids, and plasma glucose in healthy subjects", *American Journal of Clinical Nutrition*, **87**, 1262–1267; Das, S. G., and Savage, G. P. (2012) "Total and soluble oxalate content of some Indian spices", *Plant Foods for Human Nutrition*, **67(2)**, 186–190.

10. Locher, C., Frey N. A., Kirsch, I., Kossowsky, J., Meyer, A., and Gaab, J. (2017) "Is the rationale more important than deception? A randomized controlled trial of open-label placebo analgesia", *Pain*, Post Author Corrections: July 12, 2017, https://doi.org/10.1097/j.pain.0000000000001012

Chapter 6: All sorts of uses: fact or fiction?

1. Srivastava, R., and Srimal., R. C. (1985) "Modification of certain inflammation induced biochemical changes by curcumin", *Indian Journal of Medical Research*, **81**, 215–223.

2. Ghatak, N. and Basu, N. (1972) "Sodium curcuminate as an effective anti-inflammatory agent", *Indian Journal of Medical Research*, **10(3)**, 235–236.

3. Kunnumakkara, A. B., Bordoloi, D., Padmavathi, G., Monisha, J., Roy, N.K., Prasad, S., and Aggarwal, B. B. (2017) "Curcumin, the golden nutraceutical: multitargeting for multiple chronic diseases", *British Journal of Pharmacology*, **174(11)**,1325–1348.

4. Selvam, R., Subramanian, L., Gayathri, R., and Angayarkanni, N. (1995) "The anti-oxidant activity of turmeric *(Curcuma longa)*", *Journal of Ethnopharmacology*, **47(2)**, 59–67.

5. Tønnessen, H. H., De Vries, H., Karlsen, J., and van Henegouwen, G. B. (1987) "Studies on curcumin and curcuminoids IX: Investigation of the photobiological activity of curcumin using bacterial indicator systems", *Journal of Pharmaceutical Science*, **76(5)**, 371–373.

6. Nagabhushan, M., Kolpe, U., and Ramaswamy, V. (2004) "The role of dietary turmeric for the low incidence of childhood leukemia in Asian Countries", poster presented at Children with Leukemia Scientific Conference, 6–10 September 2004, http://cwl2004.powerwatch.org.uk

7. Bone, K., and Mills, S. (2013) *Principles and Practice of Phytotherapy*, 2nd edn, Churchill Livingstone Elsevier, pp.900–922.

8. Singla, V., Mouli, V. P., Garg, S. K., Rai, T., Choudhury, B. N., Verma, P., Deb, R., Tiwari, V., Rohatgi, S., Kedia, R. D. S., Sharma, P. K., Makharia, G., Ahuja, V., (2014) "Induction with NCB-02 (curcumin) enema for mild-to-moderate distal ulcerative colitis — A randomized, placebo-controlled, pilot study", *Journal of Crohn's and Colitis* **8(3)**, 208–214.

9. Baghdasaryan, A., Claudel, T., Kosters, A., Gumhold, J., Silbert, D., Thüringer, A., Leski, K., Fickert, P., Karpen, S. J., and Rauner, M. (2010) "Curcumin improves sclerosing cholangitis in Mdr2-/- mice by inhibition of cholangiocyte inflammatory response and portal myofibroblast proliferation", *Gut*, **59**, 521–530.

10. Agarwal, K. A., Tripathi, C. D., Agarwal, B. B., and Saluja, S. (2011) "Efficacy of turmeric (curcumin) in pain and postoperative fatigue after laparoscopic cholecystectomy: a double blind randomized placebo-controlled study", *Surgical Endoscopy*, **25(12)**, 3805–3810.

11. Rivera-Espinoza, Y., and Muriel, P. (2009) "Pharmacological actions of curcumin in liver diseases or damage", *Liver International,* **29(10)**,1457–1466.

12. Nabavi, S. F., Daglia, M., Moghaddam, A. H., Habtemariam, S., and Nabavi S M. (2014) "Curcumin and liver disease: from chemistry to medicine", *Comprehensive Reviews in Food Science and Food Safety,* **13**, 62–77.

13. Uchio, R., Higashi, Y., Kohama, Y., Kawasaki, K., Hirao, T., Muroyama, K., and Murosaki, S. (n.d.) "A hot water extract of turmeric (*Curcuma longa*) suppresses acute ethanol-induced liver injury in mice by inhibiting hepatic oxidative stress and inflammatory cytokine production" *Journal of Nutritional Science,* **6**, published online 12 January 2017, https://doi.org/10.1017/jns.2016.43

14. Commission E monograph on turmeric: http://cms.herbalgram.org/commissione/Monographs/Monograph0361.html

15. *Rhizoma Curcuma longa* in *WHO Monographs on Selected Medicinal Plants* – Vol. 1 http://apps.who.int/medicinedocs/en/d/Js2200e/14.html

16. Srinivasan, M. (1972) "Effect of curcumin on blood sugar seen in a diabetic subject", *Indian Journal of Medical Sciences,* **26**, 269–270.

17. Zhang, D-W., Fu, M., Gao, S-H., and Liu, J-L. (2013) "Curcumin and diabetes: a systematic review," *Evidence-Based Complementary and Alternative Medicine,* **2013**, Article ID 636053, http://dx.doi.org/10.1155/2013/636053

18. Khajehdehi, P., Pakfetrat, M., Javidnia, K., Azad, F., Malekmakan, L., Nasab, M.H., and Dehghanzadeh, G. (2011) "Oral supplementation of turmeric attenuates proteinuria, transforming growth factor-β and interleukin-8 levels in patients with overt type 2 diabetic nephropathy: a randomized, double-blind and placebo-controlled study", *Scandinavian Journal of Urology and Nephrology,* **45(5)**, 365–370.

19. Arafa, H. M. (2005) "Curcumin attenuates diet-induced hypercholesterolemia in rats," *Medical Science Monitor,* **11**, BR228–BR234.

20. Alwi, I., Santoso, T., Suyono, S., Sutrisna, B., Suyatna, F. D., Kresno, S.B., and Ernie, S. (2008) "The effect of curcumin on lipid level in patients with acute coronary syndrome", *Acta Medica Indonesiana,* **40(4)**, 201–210.

21. NCB-02 is a standardized extract of *Curcuma longa* containing 78% curcuminoids, 72% of which is curcumin, 18.08% demethoxycurcumin and 9.42% bisdemethoxycurcumin. It appears to have been used in three research studies since 2007 one of which was published by The Himalaya Drug Company which may have been producing this extract, although currently it does not appear to be commercially available.

22. Usharani, P., Mateen, A. A., Naidu, M.U., Raju, Y.S., and Chandra, N. (2008) "Effect of NCB-02, atorvastatin and placebo on endothelial function, oxidative stress and inflammatory markers in patients with type 2 diabetes mellitus: a randomized, parallel-group, placebo-controlled, 8-week study:, *Drugs in R&D*, **9(4)**, 243–250.

23. Baum, L., Cheung, S.K., Mok, V.C., Lam, L.C., Leung, V. P., Hui, E., Ng, C. C., Chow, M., Ho, P. C., Lam, S., Woo, J., Chiu, H. F., Goggins, W., Zee, B., Wong, A., Mok, H., Cheng, W. K., Fong, C., Lee, J. S., Chan, M. H., Szeto, S. S., Lui, V. W., Tsoh, J., Kwok, T. C., Chan, I. H., and Lam, C. W. (2007) "Curcumin effects on blood lipid profile in a 6-month human study", *Pharmacological Research*, **56(6)**, 509–514.

24. https://phcuk.org/eat-fat-cut-the-carbs-and-avoid-snacking-to-reverse-obesity-and-type-2-diabetes-national-obesity-forum/

25. Lopresti, A. L., Hood, S. D., and Drummond, P. D. (2012) "Multiple antidepressant potential modes of action of curcumin: a review of its anti-inflammatory, monoaminergic, antioxidant, immune-modulating and neuroprotective effects", *Journal of Psychopharmacology*, **26(12)**,1512–1524; Lopresti, A. L., Maes, M., Maker, G. L., Hood, S. D., and Drummond, P. D. (2014) "Curcumin for the treatment of major depression: a randomised, double-blind, placebo controlled study", *Journal of Affective Disorders*,**167**, 368–375.

26. http://www.prnewswire.com/news-releases/study-shows-turmeric-can-reduce-symptoms-of-depression-anxiety-546535422.html#

27. Andrade, C. (2014) "A critical examination of studies on curcumin for depression," *Journal of Clinical Psychiatry*, **75(10)**, e1110–e1112.

28. Mishra, S., and Palanivelu, K. (2008) "The effect of curcumin (turmeric) on Alzheimer's disease: an overview", *Annals of Indian Academy of Neurology*, **11(1)**, 13–19.

29. Hucklenbroich, J., Klein, R., Neumaier, B., Graf, R., Fink, G. R., Schroeter, M., and Rueger, M. A. (2014) "Aromatic-turmerone induces neural stem cell proliferation *in vitro* and *in vivo*", *Stem Cell Research & Therapy*, 5, 100.

30. Rainey-Smith, S. R., Brown, B. M., Sohrabi, H. R., Shah, H. R. T., Goozee, K. G., Gupta, V. B., and Martins, R. N. (2016) "Curcumin and cognition: a randomised, placebo-controlled, double-blind study of community-dwelling older adults", *British Journal of Nutrition*, 115, 2106–2113.

31. Ringman, J. M., Frautschy, S. A., Teng, E., Begum, A. N., Bardens, J., Beigi, M., Gylys, K. H., Badmaev, V., Heath, D. D., Apostolova, L. G., Porter, V., Vanek, Z., Marshall, G. A., Hellemann, G., Sugar, C., Masterman, D. L., Montine, T. J., Cummings, J. L., and Cole, G. M., (2012) "Oral curcumin for Alzheimer's disease: tolerability and efficacy in a 24-week randomized, double blind, placebo-controlled study", *Alzheimer's Research & Therapy*, 4(5), 43.

32. Ng, T.P., Chiam, P.C., Lee, T., Chua, H. C., Lim, L., and Kua, E.H. (2006) "Curry consumption and cognitive function in the elderly", *American Journal of Epidemiology*, 164, 898–906.

33. https://www.alzheimers.org.uk/info/20010/risk_factors_and_prevention/147/turmeric

34. Lal, B., Kapoor, A. K., Asthana, O. P., Agrawal, P. K., Prasad, R., Kumar, P., and Srimal, R. C. (1999), "Efficacy of curcumin in the management of chronic anterior uveitis", *Phytotherapy Research*, 13(4), 318–322.

35. Allegri, P., Mastromarino, A., and Neri, P. (2010) "Management of chronic anterior uveitis relapses: efficacy of oral phospholipidic curcumin treatment. Long-term follow-up", *Clinical Ophthalmology*, 4, 1201–1206.

36. "Turmeric may treat retinitis pigmentosa eye disease", https://www.fic.nih.gov/News/GlobalHealthMatters/november-december-2012/Pages/eye-institute-turmeric-retinitis-pigmentosa.aspx

37. Burgos-Morón, W., Calderón-Montaño, J. M., Salvador, J., Robles, A., and López-Lázaro, M. (2010) "The dark side of curcumin", *International Journal of Cancer*, 126, 1771–1775.

38. Vareed, S. K., Kakarala, M, Ruffin, M.T., Crowell, J. A., Normolle, D. P., Djuric, Z., and Brenner, D. E. (2008) "Pharmacokinetics

of curcumin conjugate metabolites in healthy human subjects", *Cancer Epidemiology, Biomarkers & Prevention*, **17**, 1411–1417.

39. Patel, B. B., Gupta, D., Elliott, A. A., Sengupta, V., Yu,Y., and Majumdar, A. P. N. (2010) "Curcumin targets FOLFOX-surviving colon cancer cells via inhibition of EGFRs and IGF-1R", *Anticancer Research*, **30(2)**, 319–325; Ramasamy, T. S., Ayob, A. Z., Myint, H. H. L., Thiagarajah, S., and Amini, F. (2015) "Targeting colorectal cancer stem cells using curcumin and curcumin analogues: insights into the mechanism of the therapeutic efficacy", *Cancer Cell International*, **15**, 96. http://doi.org/10.1186/s12935-015-0241-x

40. Aggarwal, B. B., Shishodia, S., Takada, Y., Banerjee, S., Newman, R.A., Bueso-Ramos, C. E., and Price, J. E. (2005) "Curcumin suppresses the Paclitaxel-induced nuclear factor-KB pathway in breast cancer cells and inhibits lung metastasis of human breast cancer in nude mice", *Clinical Cancer Reserch*, **11(20)**, 7490–7498.

41. http://www.cancerresearchuk.org/about-cancer/cancer-in-general/treatment/complementary-alternative-therapies/individual-therapies/turmeric.

42. Moghadamtousi, S. Z., Kadir, H. A., Hassandarvish, P., Tajik, H., Abubakar, S., and Zandi, K. (2014) "A review on antibacterial, antiviral, and antifungal activity of aurcumin," *BioMed Research International*, Article ID 186864. http://dx.doi.org/10.1155/2014/186864

43. Mounce, B. C., Cesaro, T., Carrau, L., Vallet, T., and Vignuzzi, M. (2017) "Curcumin inhibits Zika and chikungunya virus infection by inhibiting cell binding", *Antiviral Research*, **142**, 148–157.

44. An enveloped virus is one that has an outer wrapping or envelope. This envelope comes from the infected cell, or host, in a process called "budding off". During the budding process, newly formed virus particles become "enveloped" or wrapped in an outer coat that is made from a small piece of the cell's plasma membrane. Enveloped viruses include Herpes simplex, influenza viruses, chicken pox virus as well as Zika and chikungunya.

45. Singh, K. R., Rai, D., Yadav, D., Bhargava, A., Balzarini, J., and De Clercq, E. (2010) "Synthesis, antibacterial and antiviral properties of curcumin bioconjugates bearing dipeptide, fatty acids and folic acid", *European Journal of Medicinal Chemistry*, **45**, 1078–1086.

46. James, J. S. (1996) Curcumin: clinical trial finds no antiviral effect, *AIDS Treatment News* **242**, 1–2.

47. Assawanonda, P., and Klahan, S. O. (2010) "Tetrahydrocurcuminoid cream plus targeted narrowband UVB phototherapy for vitiligo: a preliminary randomized controlled study", *Asian Pacific Journal of Cancer Prevention*, **14**, 5753–5759.

48. Heng, M. C. Y. (2010) "Curcumin targeted signaling pathways: basis for anti-photoaging and anti-carcinogenic therapy", *International Journal of Dermatology*, **49(6)**, 608–622.

49. Vaughn, A. E., Branum, A., and Sivamani, R. K. (2016) "Effects of turmeric *(Curcuma longa)* on skin health: a systematic review of the clinical evidence", *Phytotherapy Research*, **30(8)**, 1243–1264.

50. Sonavane, K., Phillips, J., Ekshyyan, O., Moore-Medlin, T., Gill, J. R., Rong, X., Lakshmaiah, R. R., Abreo, F., Boudreaux, D., Clifford, J. L., and Nathan, C-A. O. (2012) "Topical curcumin-based cream is equivalent to dietary curcumin in a skin cancer model", *Journal of Skin Cancer*, Article ID 147863, http://dx.doi.org/10.1155/2012/147863

501. Lad, U., and Lad, V. (1994) *Ayurvedic Cooking for Self-Healing*, Ayurvedic Press, Albuquerque, New Mexico.

52. Nakayama, H., Tsuge, N., Sawada, H., Masamura, N., Yamada, S., Satomi, S., and Higashi, Y. (2014) "A single consumption of curry improved postprandial endothelial function in healthy male subjects: a randomized, controlled crossover trial", *Nutrition Journal*, **13**, 67.

53. Wongcharoen, W., Jai-aue, S., Phrommintikul, A., Nawarawong, W., Eoragidpoonpol, S., Tepsuwan, T., Sukonthasarn, A., Apaijai, N., and Chattipakorn, N. (2012) "Effects of curcuminoids on frequency of acute myocardial infarction after coronary artery bypass grafting", *American Journal of Cardiology*, **110**, 40–44.

54. Conner, E. M., and Grisham, M. B. (1996) "Inflammation, free radicals, and antioxidants", *Nutrition* **12(4)**, 274–277.

Chapter 7: Spice up your menu

1. Ng, T.P., Chiam, P.C., Lee, T., Chua, H-C., Lim, L., and Kua, E-H. (2006) "Curry consumption and cognitive function in the elderly", *American Journal of Epidemiology*, **164**, 898–906.

2. Uchio, R., Higashi, Y., Kohama, Y., Kawasaki, K., Hirao, T., Muroyama, K., and Murosaki, S. (n.d.) "A hot water extract of turmeric *(Curcuma longa)* suppresses acute ethanol-induced liver injury in mice by inhibiting hepatic oxidative stress and inflammatory cytokine production", *Journal of Nutritional Science,* **6,** published online 12 January 2017, https://doi.org/10.1017/jns.2016.43

3. Vikram, J. G. (2015) "Here's how you should make turmeric milk", *Times of India,* 30 October 2015. http://timesofindia.indiatimes.com/life-style/health-fitness/home-remedies/Heres-how-you-should-make-turmeric-milk/articleshow/47467371.cms

4. Polo, M. (c.1300) *The Travels of Marco Polo,* translated Latham, R., Folio Society edition (1968) p.195.

5. Hanbury, D. (1862) *Notes of Chinese Materia Medica,* John E. Taylor, London, p.21–22. Hanbury mentions three species of gardenia with fruits used for colouring with the Chinese drug name *zhi zi (che-tsze* in Hanbury's transliteration). *Zhi zi* is now identified as *Gardenia jasminoides* (syn. *G. grandiflora*) which Hanbury describes as imparting "a beautiful colour to silk, and that they are also used medicinally in fevers and a variety of other complaints". *Zhi zi* is used to clear heat and fire and drain damp.

6. My thanks to Ash Frisby for allowing me to share her mother's curry recipes.

7. Aga, M., Iwakia, K., Ueda, Y., Ushio, S., Masaki, N., Fukuda, S., Kimoto, T., Ikeda, M., and Kurimoto, M. (2001) "Preventive effect of *Coriandrum sativum* (Chinese parsley) on localized lead deposition in ICR mice", *Journal of Ethnopharmacology,* **77 (2–3),** 203–208.

Chapter 8: Turmeric for all

1. Mancuso, C.,and Barone, E. (2009) "Curcumin in clinical practice: myth or reality?" *Trends in Pharmacological Sciences,* **30,** 333–334.

2. Shen, L., Liu, C-C., An, C-Y, and Ji, H.-F. (2016) "How does curcumin work with poor bioavaiability? Clues from experimental and theoretical studies", *Scientific Reports,* **6,** Article number: 20872. https://doi.org/10.1038/srep20872

3. Kunnumakkara, A. B., Bordoloi, D., Padmavathi, G., Monisha, J., Roy, N.K., Prasad, S., and Aggarwal, B. B. (2017) "Curcumin, the

golden nutraceutical: multitargeting for multiple chronic diseases", *British Journal of Pharmacology*, **174(11)**,1325–1348.
4. https://clinicaltrials.gov/ct2/show/NCT01811381
5. Vikram, J. G. (2015) "Here's how you should make turmeric milk", *Times of India*, 30 October 2015. http://timesofindia.indiatimes. com/life-style/health-fitness/home-remedies/Heres-how-you-shoul d-make-turmeric-milk/articleshow/47467371.cms
6. Jacobi, J. (1988) *Paracelsus: selected writings*, Princeton University Press, New York.

Appendix 1
Useful introductions to Ayurveda include:

Frawley, D. (1989) *Ayurvedic Healing*, Passage Press, Salt Lake City.
Frawley, D. and Lad, V. (1988) *The Yoga of Herbs*, Lotus Press, Santa Fe, New Mexico.
Green, A. (2000) *The Principles of Ayurveda*, Thorsons, London.

Appendix 2
Useful introductions to Traditional Chinese Medicine include:

Ody, P. (2010) *The Chinese Medicine Bible*, Godsfield, London.
Wong, K. K. (2002) *The Complete Book of Chinese Medicine*, Cosmos, Malaysia.
Chmelik, Stefan (1999) *Chinese Herbal Secrets*, Avery Publishing, New York.

Glossary

Agni: digestive fire in Ayurveda.

Ama: accumulated toxins, undigested food and waste materials in Ayurveda.

Analgesic: a substance that relieves pain.

Anthelmintic: a substance that destroys worms.

Anti-emetic: a substance to combat nausea.

Anti-spasmodic: a substance to relieve cramps, spasms or pain in skeletal of smooth muscle.

Arteriosclerosis: build up of fatty deposits in the blood vessels leading to narrowing and hardening and associated with heart disease and strokes.

Cardioprotective: protects the heart, primarily from heart disease.

Carminative: relieves flatulence, digestive colic and gastric discomfort.

Chelate: a heterocyclic compound having a central metallic ion attached by covalent bonds to two or more non-metallic atoms in the same molecule.

Chelation: the formation of chelates – used in nutritional
therapies to remove toxic metals from the body.

Cholagogue: a substance that stimulates the flow of bile from
the gall bladder and bile ducts into the duodenum.

Choleretic: a substance that stimulates the secretion of bile
by the liver therby increaseing the flow.

Demulcent: anti-irritant; a herb rich in mucilage that
is soothing and protective to inflamed or irritable
mucous surfaces.

Depurative: a blood purifier.

Diaphoretic: a substance that increases sweating.

Diuretic: a substance that encourages urine flow.

Emmenagogue: a substance which stimulates menstruation.

Emollient: a substance which has a soothing and protective
action on the surface of the body.

Expectorant: a substance that helps to liquefy and loosen
sticky mucus making it easier to expel from the
respiratory tract by coughing.

Febrifuge: a substance that reduces fever.

Galactagogue: a substance that stimulates milk flow in
nursing mothers.

Garam masala: literally "hot spice mixture". A variable
condiment used in Indian cookery which will
typically contain black and/or white peppercorns,
cloves, cinnamon or cassia bark, mace, black and/or
green cardamom pods, bay leaf, cumin, coriander and
sometimes also small amounts of star anise, asafoetida,
chilli, and cubeb.

Haemostatic: a substance that arrests bleeding.

Hepatitis: inflammation of the liver.

Hepatoprotective: a substance that prevents damage to
the liver.

Hypoglycaemic: a substance that reduce blood sugar levels.

Hypolipdaemic: lipid lowering.

Nephroprotective: a substance that prevents damage to
     the kidneys.

Neuroprotective: a substance capable of protecting brain
     function and structure.

Oxytocic: a substance which increases uterine contractions
     during labour and also stimulates milk flow.

Rajasic: in Ayurveda, foods or herbs that promote rajas and
     in excess may lead to aggressiveness and irritability.
     They include caffeinated drinks, over-spicy foods,
     pepper, chilli and cloves.

Sattvic: in Ayurveda, foods or herbs that encourage
     sattva – clarity of mind and good health. They include
     vegetables, fruit, nuts, fresh milk, ginger, basil and
     jasmine flowers.

Stomachic: a substance that strengthens stomach function.

Tamasic: in Ayurveda, foods or herbs that encourage tamas
     and in excess have a sedative effect causing mental
     dullness and lethargy, They include meat, alcohol, stale
     food, asafoetida, garlic and valerian.

Vasodilator: a substance that dilates (makes larger)
     blood vessels.

Vasoprotective: a substance to alleviate certain conditions
     of the blood vessels such as haemorrhoids and
     varicose veins.

Vermifuge: a substance that expels worms.

Postscript

While this book has been in production inevitably new studies have been published about turmeric.

One hitting the media headlines, by researchers from the Semel Institute for Neuroscience and Human Behavior at the University of California, was a long-term (18 month) double-blind, placebo controlled trial using Theracurmin® involving 46 non-demented adults aged between 50 and 90.[1] Half the subjects were given 90mg of the curcumin supplement daily and the other half placebo and all were given brain scans at the start and end of the trial. After 18 months the curcumin group showed significant improvement in various cognitive tests while the placebo group's skills were unchanged. Those taking curcumin also had mild improvements in mood, and their brain scans showed significantly less amyloid and tau signals in the amygdala and hypothalamus than those who took placebo. According to lead researcher, Dr Garry Small "Exactly how curcumin exerts its effects is not certain, but it may be due to it ability to reduce brain inflammation, which has been linked to both Alzheimer's disease and major depression".

This trial   suggests that there may be benefits of taking regular doses or curcumin as we grow older and become more forgetful.

A second – covering a very different subject – was also notable, with researchers from Bristol University finding that turmeric's anti-parasitic properties are equally effective on dogs.[2] Dogs sprayed with turmeric oil (2.5% in water) attracted significantly fewer ticks than unsprayed dogs, or those sprayed with orange oil. Lead researcher, Penelope Goode, was "surprised at how effective turmeric was" and suggests that dog owners could make their own spray until a branded product becomes available.

Turmeric essential oil is available from commercial suppliers: add 2.5ml to 100ml of water in a spray bottle, shake the bottle well and use that to spray your dog's stomach and legs where ticks are most likely to attach.

Notes

1   Small, G. W., Siddarth, P., Li, Z., Miller, K. J., Ercoli, L., Emerson, N. D., Martinmez, J., Wong, K-P., Liu, J., Merrill, D. A., Chen, S. T., Henning, S. M., Satyamurthy, N., Huang, S-C., Heber, D., and Barrio, J. R. (2018) "Memory and brain amyloid and tau effects of a bioavailable form of curcumin in non-demented adults: a double-blind, placebo-controlled 18-month trial", in *American Journal of Geriatric Psychiatry*, **26(3)**, 266–277.

2   Goode, P., Ellse, L., and Wall., R. (n.d.) "Preventing tick attachment to dogs using essential oils" in *Tick and Tick-borne Diseases*, published online 27 March 2018, https://doi.org/10.1016/j.ttbdis.2018.03.029